Surgery
IN*focus*

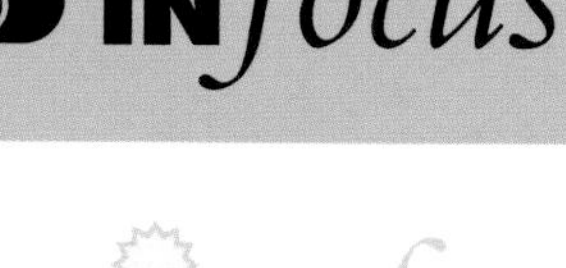

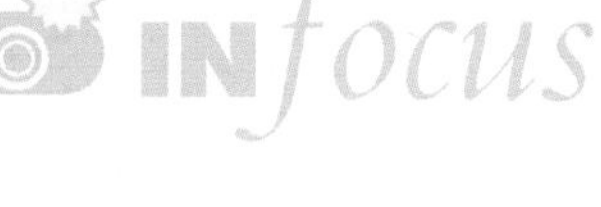
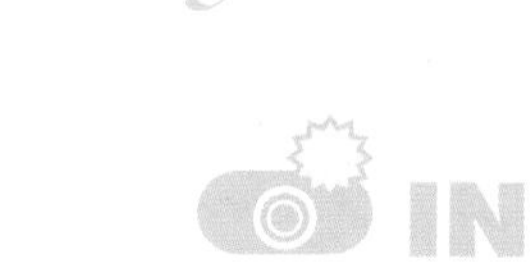
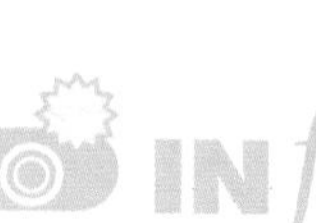
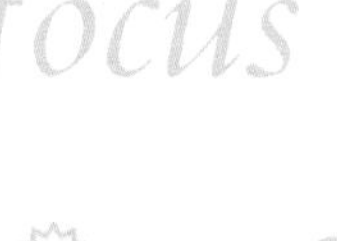
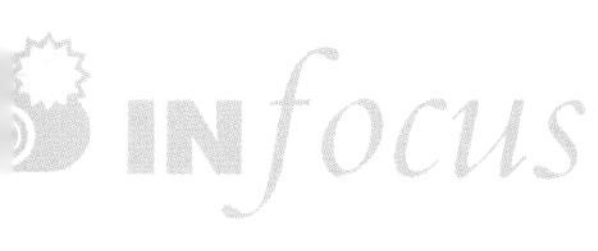
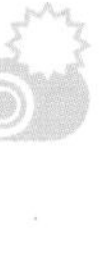
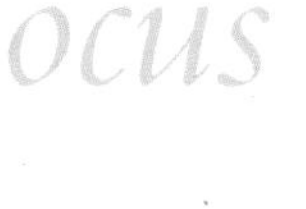
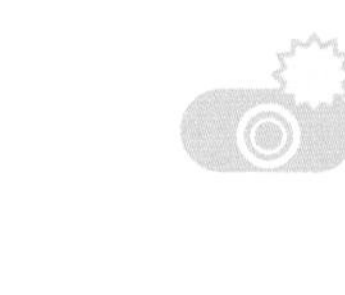

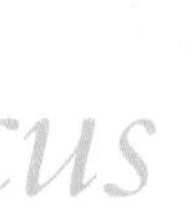

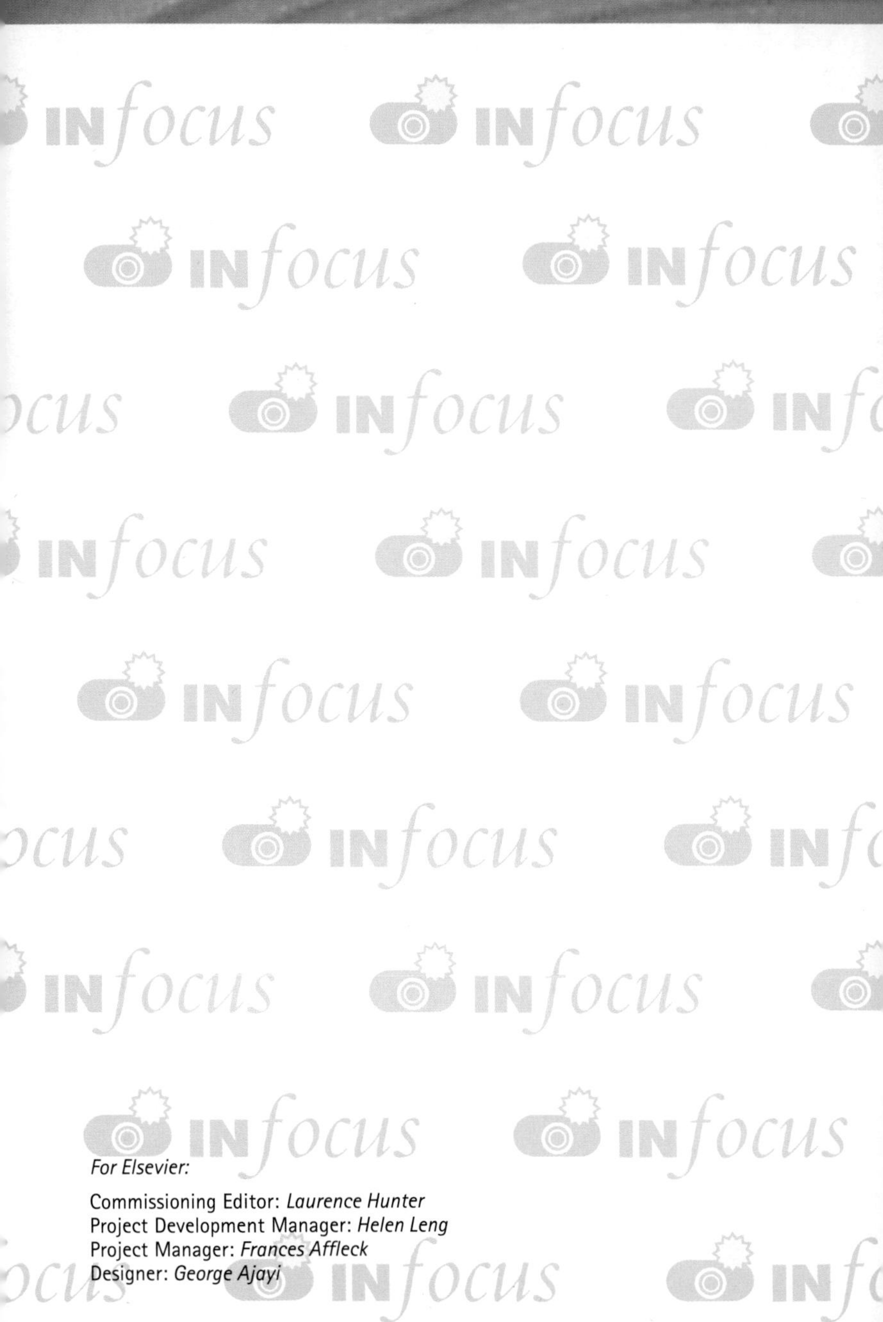

For Elsevier:

Commissioning Editor: *Laurence Hunter*
Project Development Manager: *Helen Leng*
Project Manager: *Frances Affleck*
Designer: *George Ajayi*

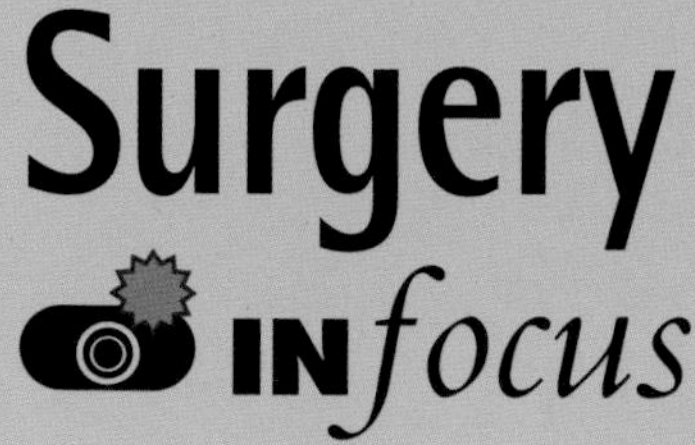

Rowan W Parks MD FRCSI FRCSEd

Senior Lecturer in Surgery
Department of Clinical & Surgical Sciences
University of Edinburgh
Royal Infirmary of Edinburgh
Edinburgh
UK

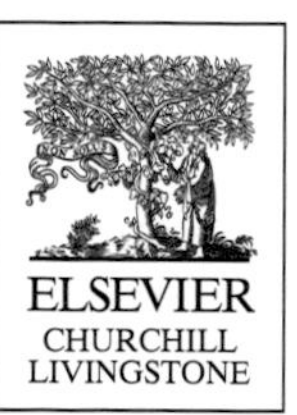

EDINBURGH LONDON NEW YORK OXFORD PHILADELPHIA ST LOUIS SYDNEY TORONTO 2005

ELSEVIER | CHURCHILL LIVINGSTONE
An imprint of Elsevier Limited

First edition 2005

ISBN 0443073775

British Library Cataloguing in Publication Data
A catalogue record for this book is available from the British Library

Library of Congress Cataloging in Publication Data
A catalog record for this book is available from the Library of Congress

Note
Medical knowledge is constantly changing. Standard safety precautions must be followed, but as new research and clinical experience broaden our knowledge, changes in treatment and drug therapy may become necessary or appropriate. Readers are advised to check the most current product information provided by the manufacturer of each drug to be administered to verify the recommended dose, the method and duration of administration, and contraindications. It is the responsibility of the practitioner, relying on experience and knowledge of the patient, to determine dosages and the best treatment for each individual patient. Neither the publisher nor the author assumes any liability for any injury and/or damage to persons or property arising from this publication.

Printed in China

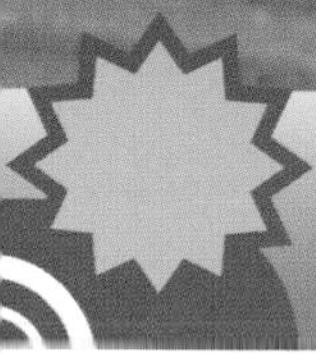

Acknowledgements

I am indebted to Mr Donald Greig (Consultant Surgeon, Hong Kong) and Professor James Garden (Regius Professor of Surgery Edinburgh) who contributed a significant number of clinical images for this publication. I am also indebted to the following who have provided images: Mr John Forsythe (Consultant Surgeon, Edinburgh); Mr Trevor Crofts (Consultant Surgeon, Edinburgh); Ms Anna Paisley (Specialist Registrar, Edinburgh); Professor George Parks (Retired Consultant Surgeon, Belfast); Mr Simon Paterson-Brown (Consultant Surgeon, Edinburgh); Mr Michael Dixon (Consultant Surgeon, Edinburgh); Professor Andrew Bradbury (Professor of Vascular Surgery, Birmingham); Mr James Mander (Consultant Surgeon, Edinburgh); Dr Doris Redhead (Consultant Radiologist, Edinburgh) and Dr Hamish Ireland (Consultant Radiologist, Edinburgh).

I am grateful for the guidance and encouragement from Ms Helen Leng and Mr Laurence Hunter from Elsevier and I trust that the completed book will be a useful addition to the In Focus series. I am indebted to Susan Keggie, my university secretary, for her hard work and secretarial expertise.

Finally, I would like to thank my wife Janet and children Matthew, Amy, Naomi and Thomas for their amazing tolerance and unwavering support for this project and my other academic endeavours.

Contents

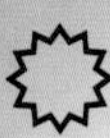

1 Benign infective epidermal lesions

Viral infection

- Human papilloma virus (common wart)
- Pox virus (molluscum contagiosum)
- Herpes virus (herpes simplex, herpes zoster)

Clinical features

Cutaneous warts are common and are most prevalent in children. They are most frequently found on the hands and fingers, or may affect the sole of the foot (plantar warts). They form greyish-brown, round or oval elevated lesions with a filiform surface and keratinized projections. Plantar warts may cause considerable pain.

Molluscum contagiosum consists of individual smooth, dome-shaped lesions that have a characteristic central depression or umbilication; if squeezed a central white core called the molluscum body can be expressed.

Management

Warts grow and regress spontaneously over several months but they often require treatment to relieve pain, irritation or inconvenience. Keratolytic applications or cryotherapy (application of liquid nitrogen) is often the first choice of treatment. Physical abrasion of warts can be achieved by curettage, diathermy or laser therapy.

Bacterial infection

Cellulitis is a diffuse spreading infection of the subcutaneous tissues and deeper layers of the skin (Fig. 1). Causative organisms are staphylococci, streptococci and occasionally Gram-negative rods. Erysipelas is caused by beta-haemolytic streptococci. The organisms usually gain entry via a traumatic or surgical wound.

Clinical features

The skin is thickened, red, hot and tender. The margins are fairly clearly demarcated from adjacent normal skin. There may be red lines leading proximally as a consequence of lymphangitis (Fig. 2) and the regional lymph nodes may be swollen and tender (lymphadenitis). Systemic features such as fever and tachycardia indicate bacteraemia or septicaemia.

Management

Appropriate antibiotics – penicillin for streptococci, flucloxacillin for staphylococci. Hospital admission for intravenous administration of antibiotics and analgesia may be required.

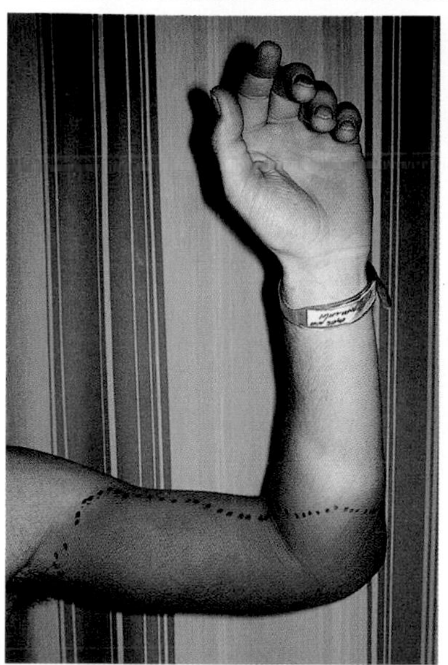

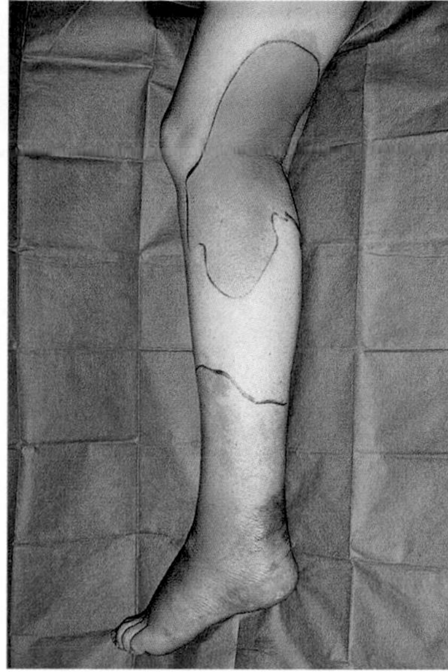

A B

Fig. 1 Cellulitis affecting (A) the upper limb; (B) the lower limb.

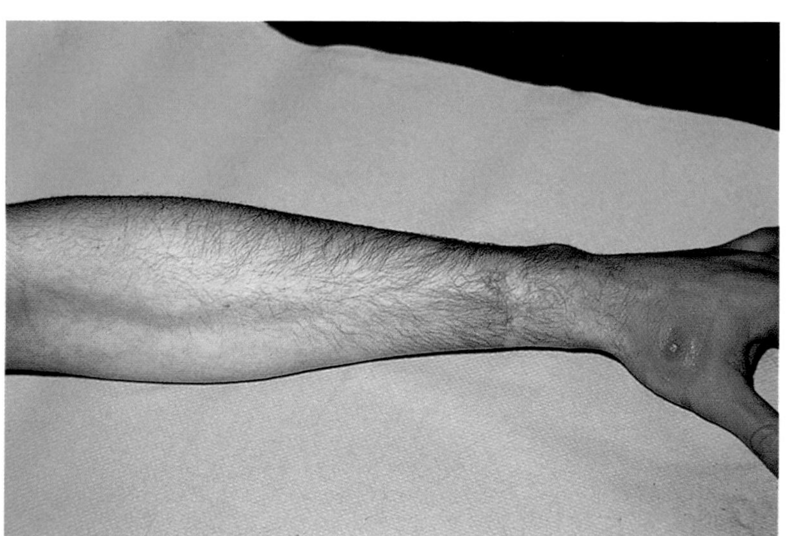

Fig. 2 Lymphangitis associated with a lesion on the dorsum of the hand.

2 Benign epidermal tumours

Classification

- Pedunculated papilloma (skin tag)
- Seborrhoeic wart (basal cell papilloma)
- Keratoacanthoma (molluscum sebaceum)

Skin tags

Clinical features

Commonly found in sites where skin surfaces rub together and the skin is therefore chronically irritated. There is a loose connective tissue core covered by epidermis, which is variably pigmented.

Skin tags appear as warty masses that hang on a stalk of surrounding normal epithelium. They may cause an itch or bleed secondary to irritation by clothing.

Management

Excision under local anaesthesia.

Seborrhoeic warts (basal cell papilloma)

Clinical features

Commonly arise on the trunk and face; may grow up to several centimetres in diameter. Lesions are raised, sharply demarcated and plaque-like with varying amounts of pigmentation. This surface is waxy with superficial clefting and fissuring (Fig. 3).

Management

Differential diagnosis of deeply pigmented papillomas from malignant melanoma can be difficult and if there is doubt excision biopsy is indicated. Otherwise, shearing back the lesion or curettage and cautery gives a satisfactory cosmetic result.

Keratoacanthoma

A nodular, usually solitary skin lesion with an irregular skin crater containing keratotic debris. The importance of this benign lesion is that it can be difficult to distinguish clinically or even histologically from squamous carcinoma. It usually grows rapidly over 4–6 weeks and then enters a static phase, which may last 3–4 months before spontaneous resolution (Fig. 4).

Management

Excision of the lesion if there is diagnostic doubt, but it may also be eradicated by curettage.

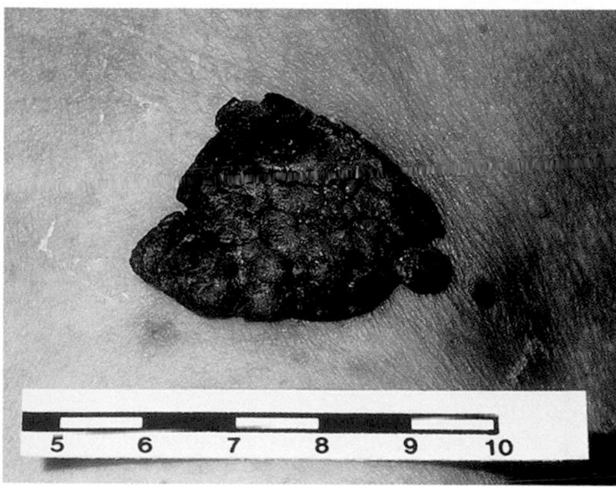

Fig. 3 Seborrhoeic keratosis.

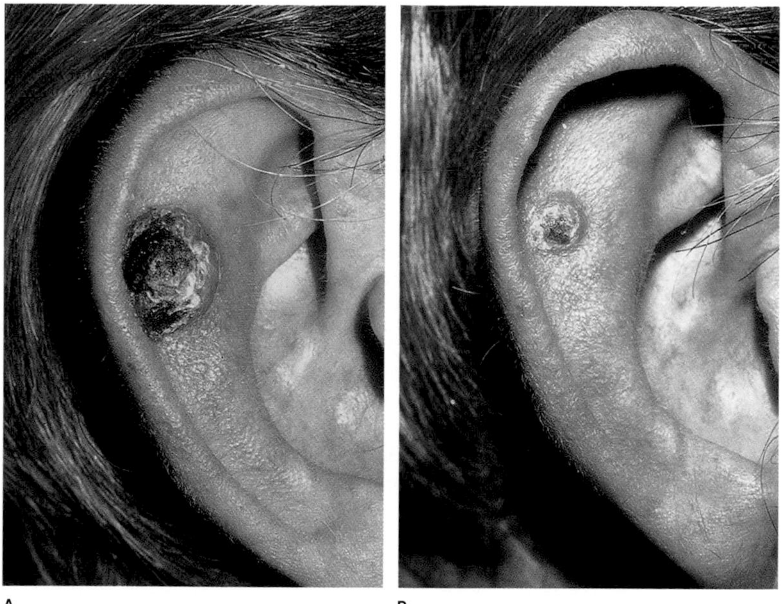

A

B

Fig. 4 Keratoacanthoma (A) at presentation; (B) 4 weeks later, after spontaneous regression.

3 Malignant epidermal lesions

Classification

There are two clinical types of carcinoma, both of which arise from keratinocytes:

- Basal cell carcinoma
- Squamous-cell carcinoma

Predisposing factors

- Exposure to sunlight
- Immunosuppression
- Chemical carcinogens, e.g. arsenic, tar and soot
- Chronic ulceration, e.g. chronic leg ulcers, old burns, tuberculosis of the skin
- Hereditary conditions, e.g. xeroderma pigmentosum
- Exposure to radiation

Clinical features

Basal cell carcinomas begin as translucent or pearly-white nodules with visible telangiectatic blood vessels. Lesions may ulcerate, bleed and then heal again but as they enlarge they form irregular ulcers (rodent ulcers; Fig. 5). Characteristically, they cause local invasion and destruction of surrounding tissues (Fig. 6) but rarely metastasize.

Squamous-cell carcinoma usually present as an enlarging, painless ulcer with a rolled, indurated margin or may have a proliferative, exophytic, cauliflower-like appearance with areas of ulceration, bleeding or serous exudation (Fig. 7). Squamous-cell carcinomas invade locally, may spread to regional lymph nodes and occasionally metastasize to distant areas.

Management

Malignant epidermal lesions should be excised. Local radiotherapy may be appropriate for selected lesions depending on the tumour size, site and aggressiveness. Palpable lymph nodes are an indication for regional lymphadenectomy by block dissection. This may be followed by adjuvant radiotherapy.

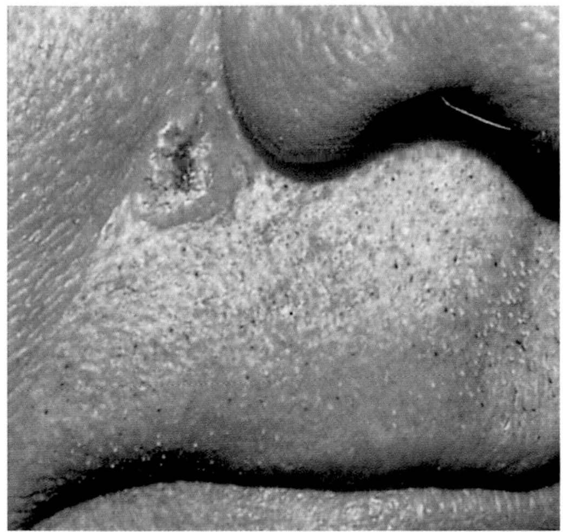

Fig. 5 Basal cell carcinoma affecting the nasolabial fold.

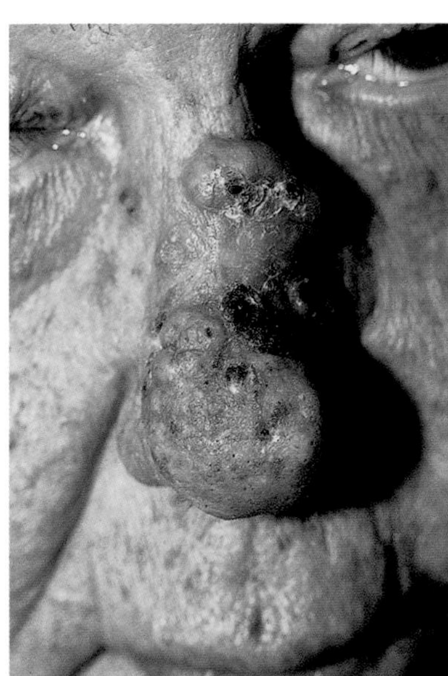

Fig. 6 Extensive basal cell carcinoma of the nose.

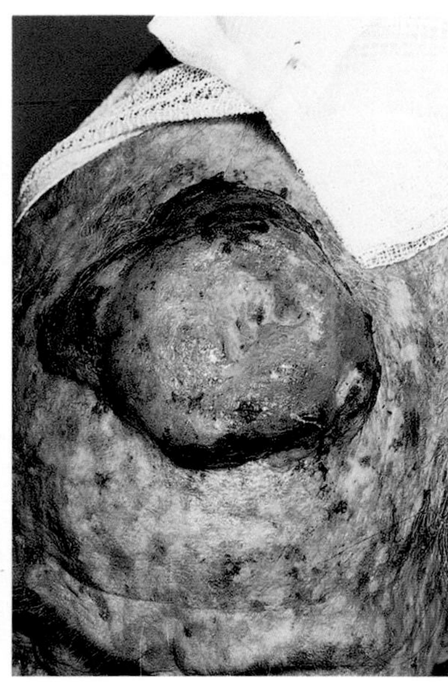

Fig. 7 Squamous-cell carcinoma involving the scalp.

4 Skin lesions of vascular origin

Classification

- Campbell de Morgan spots
- Spider naevi
- Haemangioma (capillary, cavernous)
- Port wine stains
- Strawberry naevi

Clinical features

Campbell de Morgan spots appear as small, cherry-coloured capsules on the trunk. They are very common and of no significance, but may become increasingly numerous with age.

Spider naevi or telangiectasiae consist of a central arteriole from which radiate dilated capillaries (Fig. 8). Isolated spider naevi may be found in normal individuals but more than five usually indicates liver cirrhosis. Localized treatment is rarely required.

Haemangiomas are congenital haematomas, which may give rise to salmon-pink discoloration of the skin. Variants include the port-wine stain on the face, neck or scalp (Fig. 9). They cause considerable cosmetic distress. Surgical treatment is rarely successful. Argon laser treatment may provide good results in some patients; however, covering cosmetics are frequently required.

Strawberry naevi may appear in infancy and grow with age. They are usually bright red fleshy lesions (Fig. 10). Spontaneous involution occurs and they usually disappear, leaving no scar.

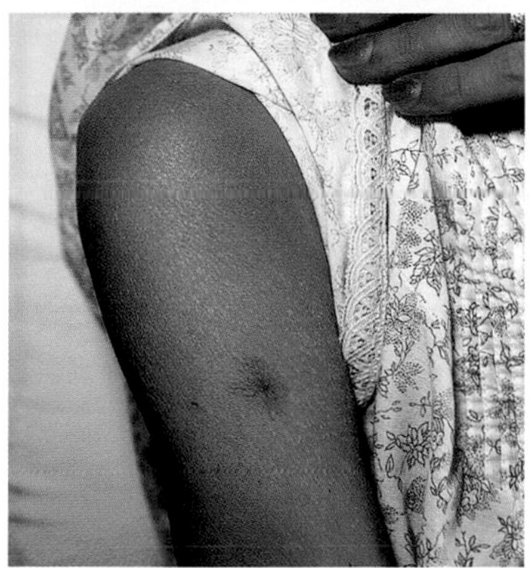

Fig. 8 Spider naevus in a patient with cirrhosis of the liver.

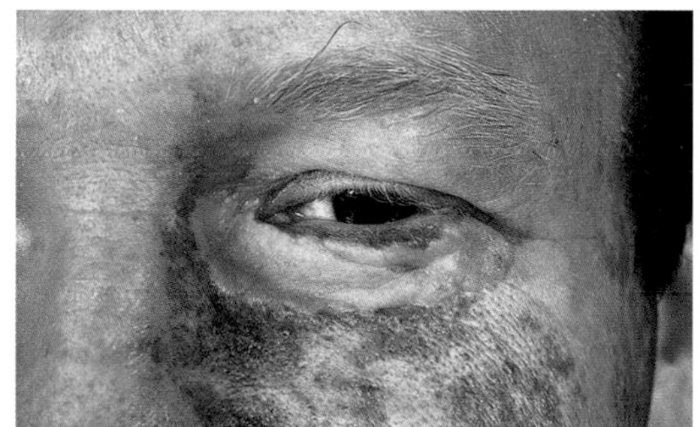

Fig. 9 Capillary haemangioma.

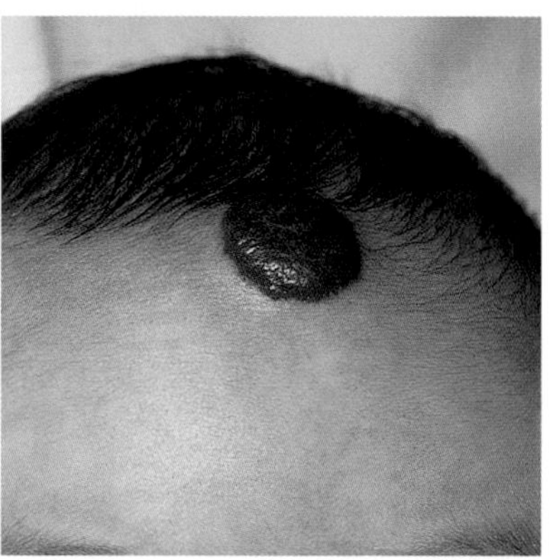

Fig. 10 Strawberry naevus of the forehead.

5 Pigmented skin lesions

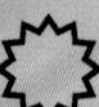

Classification

- Benign naevi (junctional, intradermal, compound, blue, juvenile)
- Malignant melanoma

Clinical features

Benign melanocytic naevi (common moles) have a flat or slightly raised brown/black appearance and are covered by normal epidermis (Fig. 11). They may grow during childhood but usually become quiescent at puberty and may later atrophy.

The giant hairy naevus (Fig. 12) is present at birth and may cover a large area.

Malignant melanomas predominately affect fair-skinned individuals (Fig. 13). Exposure to sunlight is the key aetiological factor. Half of all malignant melanomas arise in a pre-existing naevus. Malignant melanomas invade the dermis and spread rapidly via the lymphatic system and the bloodstream.

Melanomas may be classified as growing radially (superficial spreading type; Fig. 14) or vertically (nodular type). Most malignant melanomas are black or dark brown, flat or nodular lesions, which may bleed or ulcerate. If a pre-existing or new mole enlarges, darkens, bleeds or becomes inflamed, ulcerated or itchy it should be excised.

Prognostic factors

Tumour thickness on histological examination (Breslow depth) is the most useful guide to prognosis and has proved more accurate than the level of invasion (Clark's levels). Other factors affecting prognosis include:

- Pathological stage
- Presence of satellite lesions
- Presence of ulceration
- Number and size of lymph node metastases
- Sex – males fare worse than females

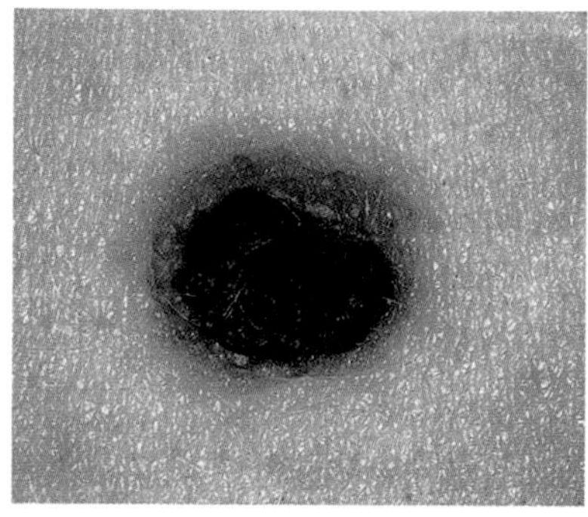

Fig. 11 Melanocytic naevus. This lesion appears particularly on the face and trunk.

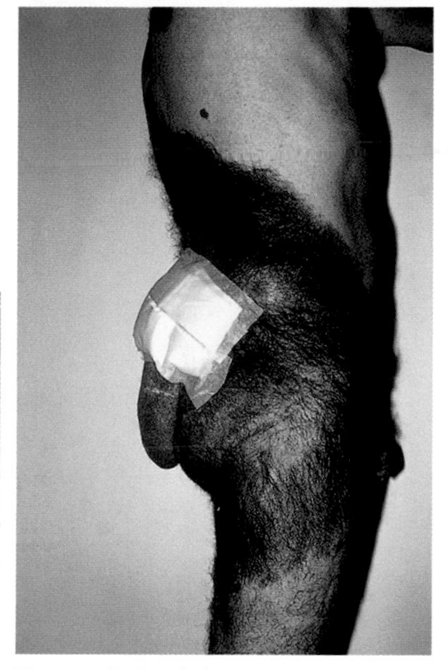

Fig. 12 A giant hairy naevus.

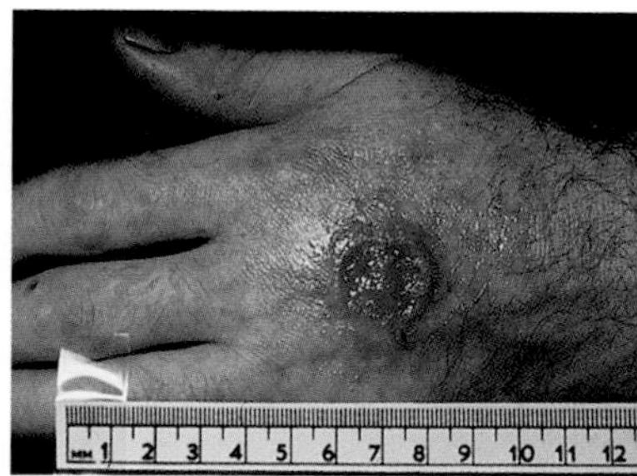

Fig. 13 Amelanotic melanoma.

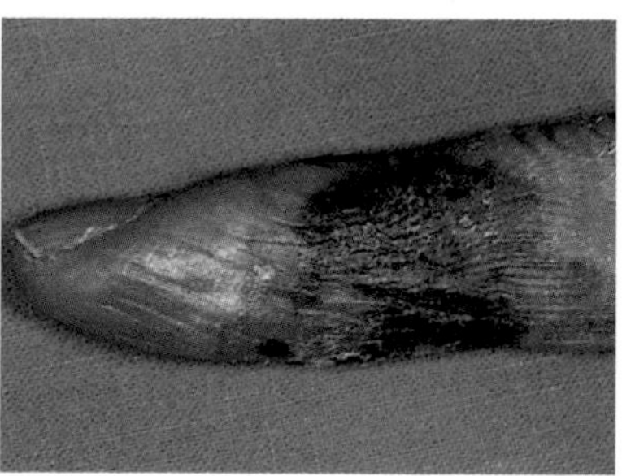

Fig. 14 Superficial spreading melanoma.

6 Miscellaneous skin lesions

Lipoma

A benign tumour of fat that varies in size from 1 to 20 cm (Fig. 15). The overlying skin is normal and easily moveable. The consistency is soft and almost fluctuant. Lipomas are removed if they are inconvenient, unsightly or very large, because of the risk of malignancy.

Pyogenic granuloma

A common inflammatory lesion of the skin, which arises following minor trauma. They are most common on the hands, feet and lips and give rise to a mass of exuberant granulation tissue containing numerous polymorphs. In spite of their name, they are not infective.

Clinical features

Solitary, firm reddish/blue fleshy nodules which may be polypoid. They are occasionally painful. The surface may be ulcerated and may bleed.

Management

Excision with curettage and cautery of the base to prevent recurrence.

Neurofibroma

These are benign tumours arising from the supporting fibroblasts of peripheral nerves. The usual appearance is of a solitary sessile or pedunculated lesion in the region of a peripheral nerve. The autosomal dominantly inherited syndrome called neurofibromatosis (von Recklinghausen's disease) is characterized by multiple neurofibromas and café-au-lait spots (Fig. 16).

Secondary (metastatic) carcinoma

Metastatic tumour deposits may present as small, hard, painless nodules in the skin (Figs 17, 18). Treatment is by local excision, radiotherapy or chemotherapy depending on the severity of symptoms and the size, number and location of secondaries.

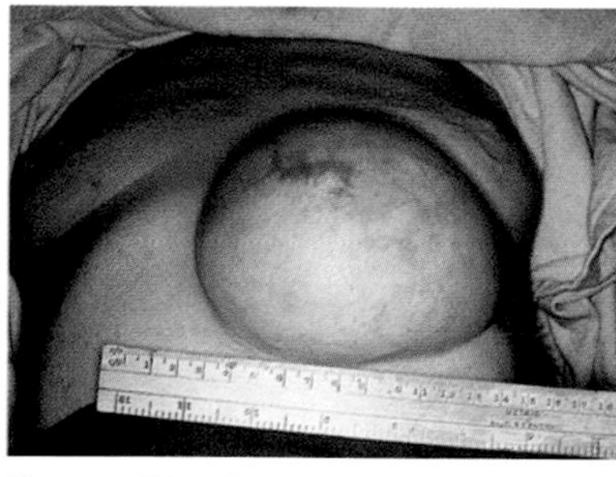

Fig. 15 Giant lipoma with sarcomatous change.

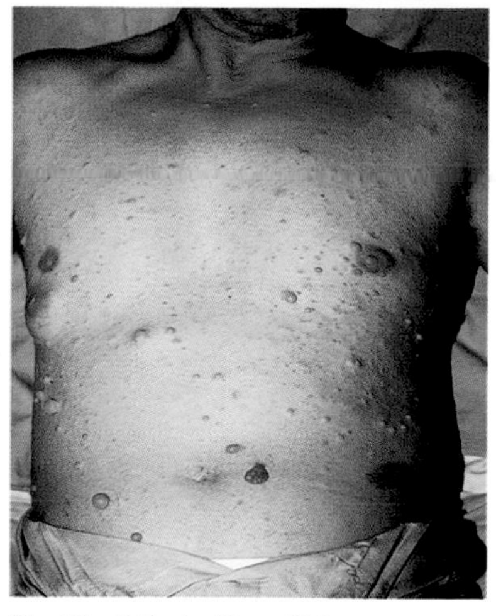

Fig. 16 Patient with multiple neurofibromata characteristic of von Recklinghausen's disease.

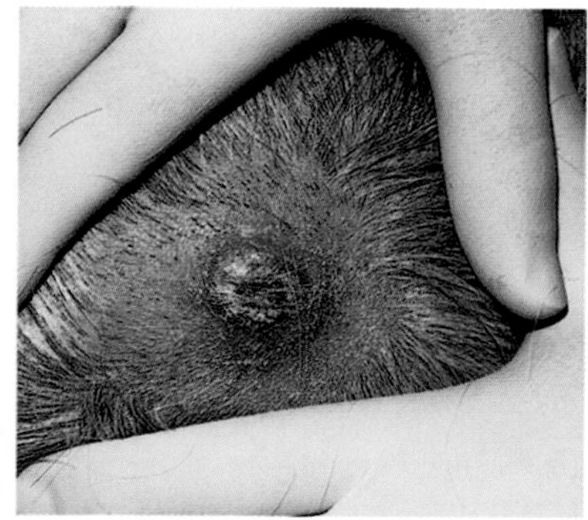

Fig. 17 Skin metastasis in scalp originating from primary pancreatic carcinoma.

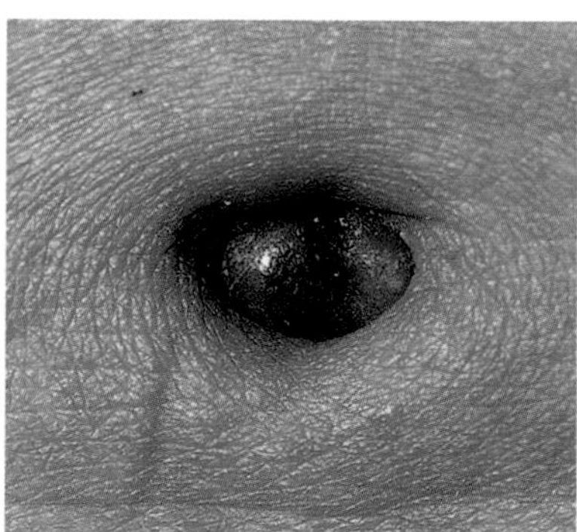

Fig. 18 Sister Joseph's nodule.

7 Skin cysts

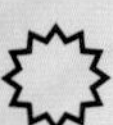

Classification

- Secondary to obstruction (epidermal cysts and pilar cysts)
- Congenital (e.g. dermoid cysts)
- Traumatic (e.g. implantation dermoids)

Epidermal cyst

These common skin lesions consist of an epithelium-lined cavity filled with viscous or semi-solid epithelial degradation products (Fig. 19). Epidermal cysts were previously described incorrectly as 'sebaceous cysts'.

Clinical features

They are usually solitary. They may be found anywhere in the body (expect the palms or soles) but are most common on the scalp, trunk, face and neck. They are smooth, rounded and covered by normal epidermis in which a blocked duct (punctum) may be visible. On palpation they have a doughy, fluctuant consistency and are usually non-tender. They originate in the skin and are attached to it but are mobile over deeper tissues.

Epidermal cysts may become traumatized, causing the contents to escape into the surrounding tissues and exciting an intense inflammatory response. This may manifest with pain, swelling, redness and discharge of liquefied cyst contents. Secondary bacterial infection may also occur (Fig. 20).

Management

Uninfected cysts are excised. Care must be taken not to puncture or to rupture the cyst to prevent recurrence. If the lesion has become inflamed then the contents are best drained and the inflammation left to subside, at which point the cyst can be excised.

Dermoid cyst

These congenital cysts are rare and arise from abnormalities of development where epithelial remnants occur. They are commonly found in the midline of the neck, scalp and face (Fig. 21). The contents of the cyst include hair, sebaceous glands and other ectodermal structures in addition to keratin. Treatment is by excision.

Implantation dermoid

In this condition a usually insignificant injury drives a fragment of dermis into the subdermal layer, from where its secretions all escape. They are most often seen on the fingers.

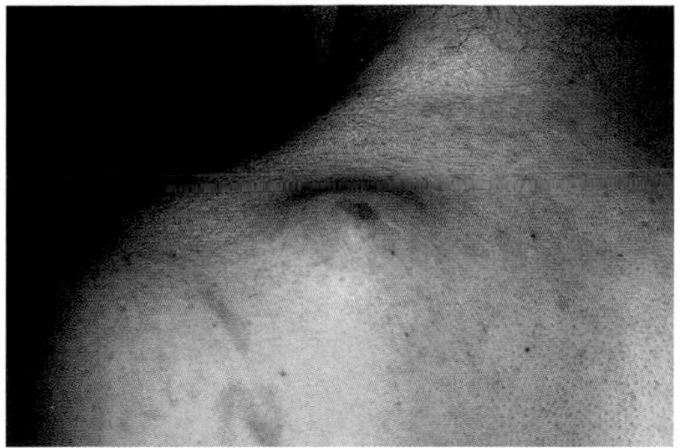

Fig. 19 Epidermal cyst in the left shoulder region of a middle-aged man.

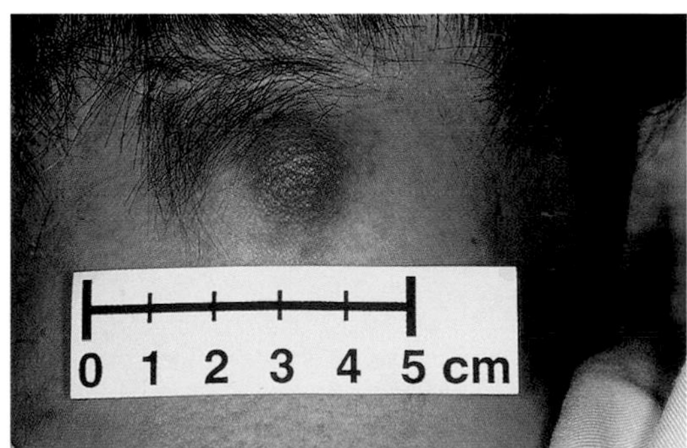

Fig. 20 Infected epidermal cyst.

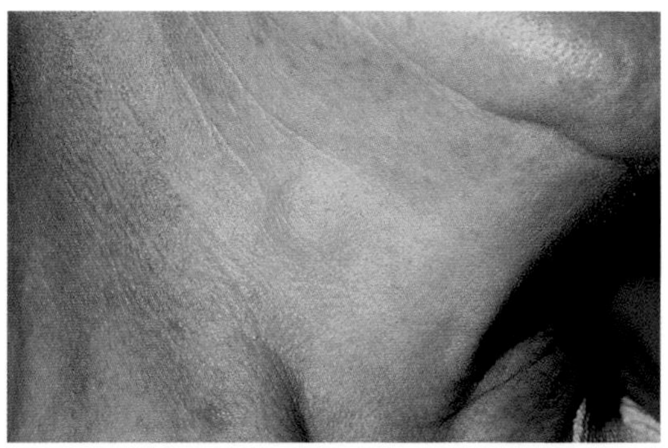

Fig. 21 Dermoid cyst in the neck.

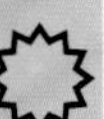

8 Ganglion

Ganglions are tense cysts containing viscous, jelly-like material. They are derived from the lining of a synovial joint, tendon sheath or are embryological remnants of synovial tissue. The cystic space does not usually communicate with the associated joint or tendon sheath.

Clinical features

Ganglia present as superficial swellings, usually about 1–2 cm in diameter. They most often occur on the dorsum of the wrist (Figs 22, 23) but may also be found in the hand and in the foot. They are rarely painful but may cause cosmetic embarrassment and occasionally mechanical limitation.

Management

The traditional treatment for a ganglion is a sharp blow with a family Bible. Aspiration of the ganglion followed by steroid injection may be used but recurrence is common. Excision of the ganglia is most effective, although recurrence may still occur.

Trigger finger

Localized thickening of the flexor tendon of a digit results in the finger catching in flexion. This is due to a thickened part of the tendon being unable to pass smoothly under the entrance to a synovial sheath at the base of the finger. Surgical treatment is the only option.

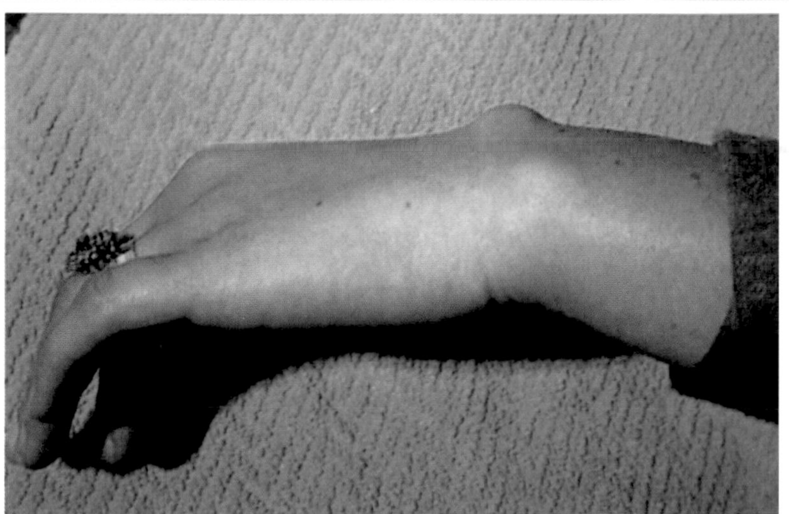

Fig. 22 Ganglion of the wrist.

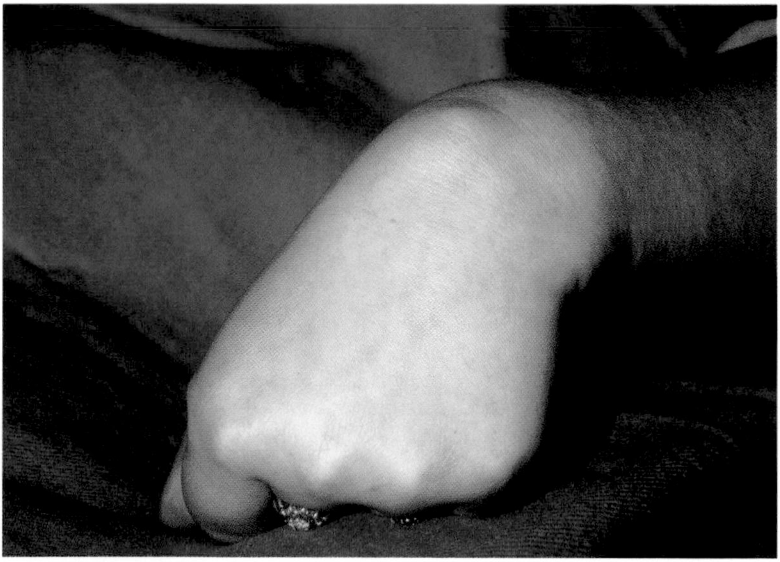

Fig. 23 Ganglion of the wrist.

9 Dupuytren's contracture

This is a condition of the hand in which there is thickening and contraction of the palmar aponeurosis.

Aetiology

Recognized associated factors include:

- Family history
- Male sex
- Excess alcohol consumption
- Diabetes mellitus
- Phenytoin therapy
- Trauma

Clinical features

Contracture is bilateral in 45%. Similar lesions occur in the plantar aponeurosis in 5%. The penile fascia is affected in 3% (Peyronie's disease). Signs are easily apparent at the base of the little and ring fingers. As the lesion progresses, the fingers gradually developed a fixed flexion deformity (Fig. 24).

Management

Several operative techniques are available. The choice depends on the extent of the lesion, the degree of disability and whether previous surgical operations have been attempted.

- Division of fibrous bands through percutaneous stab wounds
- Excision of thickened areas of fascia
- Complete fasciectomy with or without excision of the palmar skin and skin grafting
- Amputation of a single digit

Ulnar nerve injury

This is usually due to acute or chronic trauma, osteo- or rheumatoid arthritis. There is pain in the forearm and wasting of the small muscles of the hand leading, in the worst cases, to an ulnar 'claw' hand (Fig. 25). There may be reduced sensation in the ulnar distribution of the hand. The diagnosis may be made clinically, but electrophysiology is recommended to confirm the diagnosis. Treatment consists of surgically decompressing the nerve.

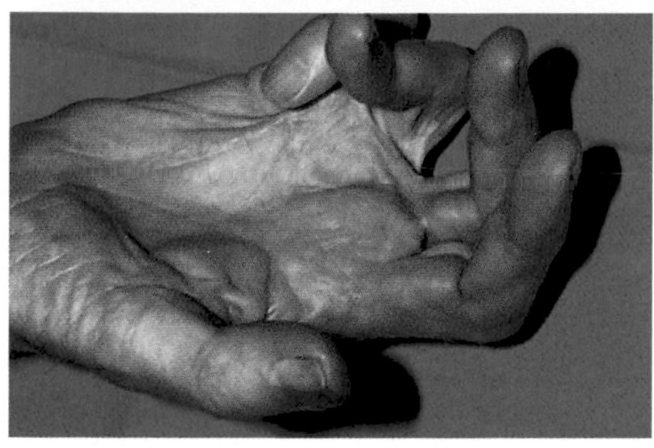

Fig. 24 Dupuytren's contracture, predominantly affecting the ring and little finger.

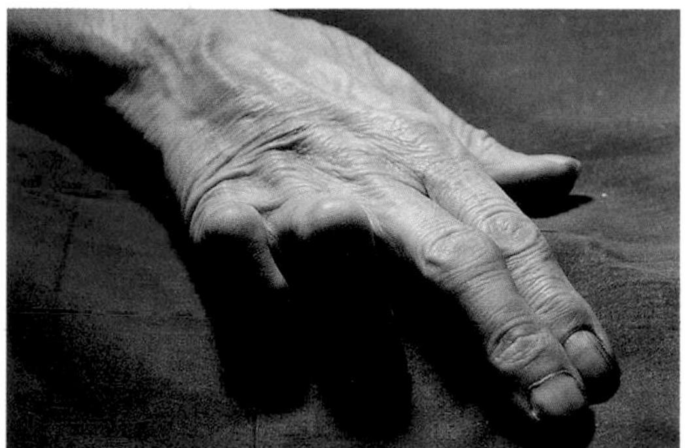

A

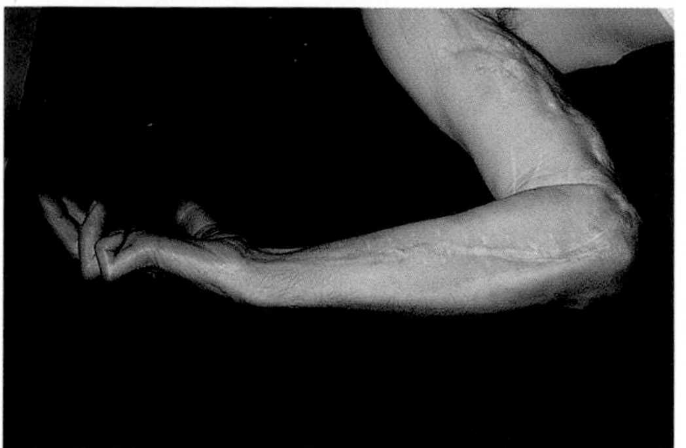

B

Fig. 25 'Claw' hand due to **(A)** ulnar nerve palsy; **(B)** previous trauma to forearm.

10 Hidradenitis suppurativa

Hidradenitis suppurativa is a chronic recurrent inflammatory process involving apocrine sweat glands and adjacent connective tissue.

Clinical features

Classically, the axillary and inguinoperineal regions are the most commonly affected areas (Figs 26, 27). It is generally thought that occlusion of the apocrine or follicular ducts by keratinous plugging leads to ductal obstruction and stasis with subsequent secondary bacterial infection. Hidradenitis suppurativa initially presents with deep-seated nodules, which tend to coalesce and may become infected, resulting in acute abscesses. These may temporarily resolve or alternatively may progress, ultimately culminating in chronic sepsis with sinus and fistula formation, multiple abscesses, persistent pain and dermal scarring. Malodorous discharge may be thin and serous or frankly purulent in nature.

Perianal hidradenitis may present with pain, swelling, purulent discharge, pruritus or bleeding and can mimic several common problems such as furunculosis, pilonidal disease, perianal abscess or Crohn's disease.

Management

- Medical treatment – antibiotics, topical synthetic retinoids, intralesional administration of triamcinolone, immunotherapy
- Conservative surgery – local incision and drainage of individual purulent lesions
- Deroofing of sinuses and fistular tracts
- Limited local excision with primary closure
- Radical surgery with wide clearance of apocrine glandular zone and subsequent skin grafting.

Prognosis

The extent of skin excision may influence recurrence rates more than a particular method of wound management.

- Recurrence after surgery is likely if excision is inadequate or if there is an unusually wide distribution of apocrine glands
- Revisional surgery is often required.

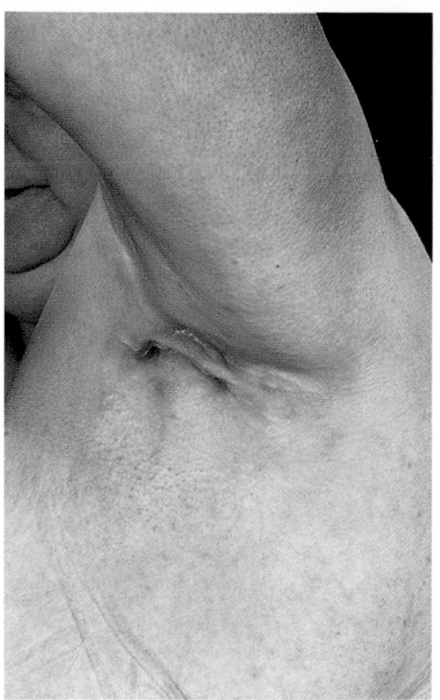

Fig. 26 Hidradenitis suppurativa affecting the left axilla.

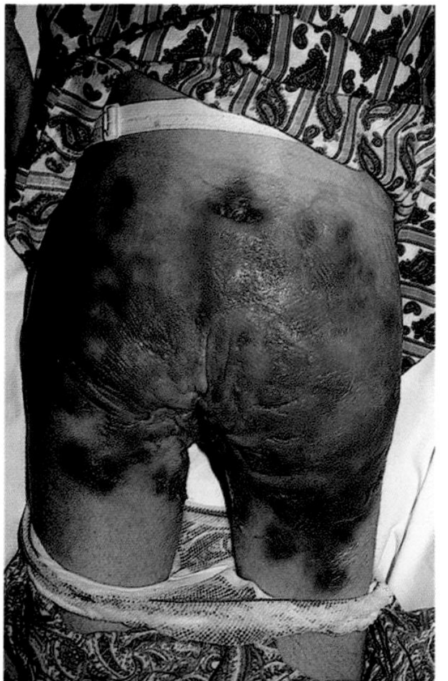

Fig. 27 Extensive hidradenitis suppurativa affecting the perineum.

11 Burns

Incidence

Approximately 12 000 hospital admissions annually in England and Wales are due to burn injuries. A third of burns occur in the home, with the rest largely occupation-related.

Classification

- Superficial partial-thickness
- Deep-partial thickness (Fig. 28)
- Full-thickness (Fig. 29)

Clinical features

In its least severe form the dermal inflammatory response consists of capillary dilatation as in the erythema of sunburn. Collection of plasma beneath coagulated epidermis results in blistering, which may be excruciatingly painful. In full thickness burns the epidermis and dermis are converted into a coagulum of dead tissue known as eschar (Fig. 30).

Complications

- Fluid loss, hypovolaemia
- Myocardial depression
- Oedema – airway obstruction, compartment syndromes
- Airway burn – hypoxia
- Haemolysis
- Sepsis – both local and generalized
- Tissue damage – myoglobinuria

Management

- First aid – arrest the burning process, protect airway
- Fluid management – e.g. volume (ml/24 h) = 4 × weight (kg) × percentage of total body surface area burned
- Pain control
- Support if organ failure – respiratory, renal
- Nutritional management
- Skin grafting
- Escharotomy (incision of eschar) if there is evidence of restricted blood flow or respiratory movement due to circumferential burns of the limbs or thorax.

Prognosis

- Age – infants and elderly fare less well
- Extent of the burn – hypovolaemic shock is anticipated if more than 15% burn in adults (10% in children)
- Depth of burn – superficial burns should heal without scarring within 3 weeks. Deep dermal burns may take longer and produce hypertrophic scarring. Full-thickness burns inevitably become infected unless excised early
- Site of burn – burns involving the face (Fig. 31), neck, hands or perineum are particularly liable to threaten appearance or function
- Associated respiratory injury – inhalation of smoke from burning plastic and foam upholstery may be fatal

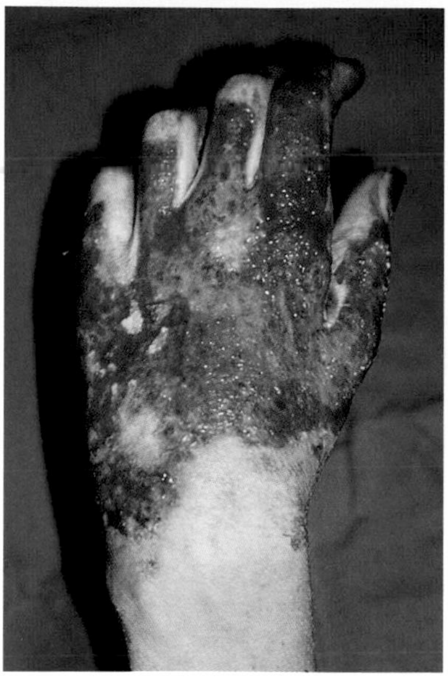

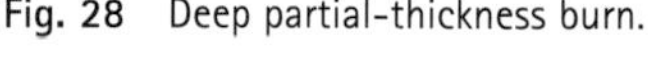

Fig. 28 Deep partial-thickness burn.

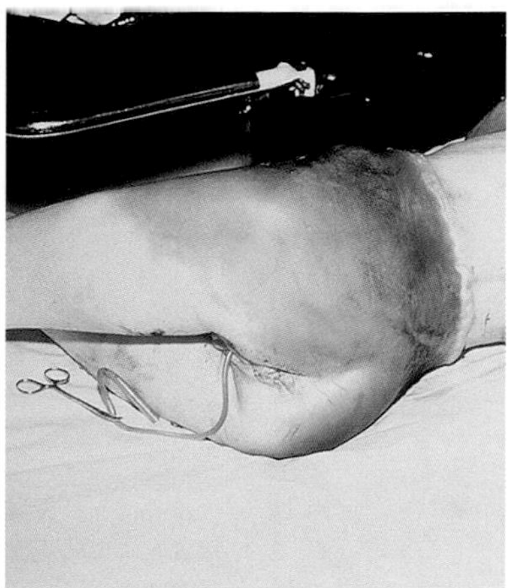

Fig. 29 Full-thickness burn.

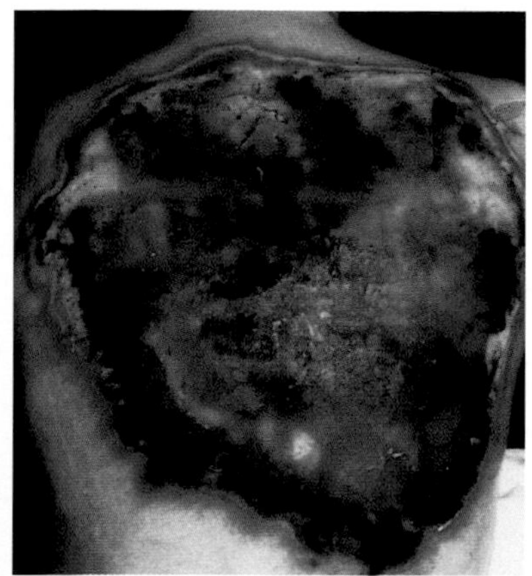

Fig. 30 Eschar involving the back. Escharotomy may be required if chest movement is restricted because of the burned tissue.

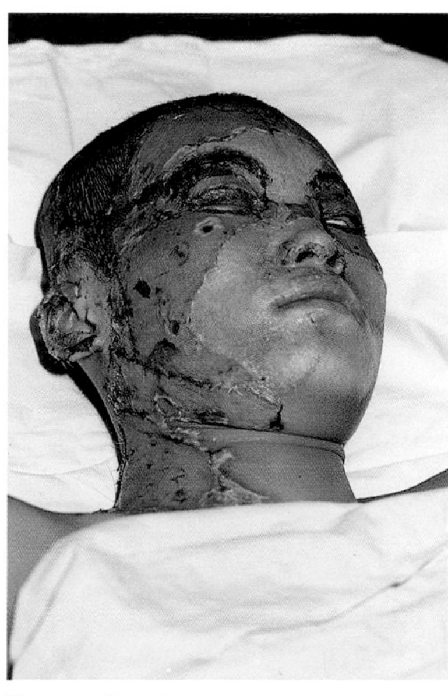

Fig. 31 Chemical burn to face.

12 Ingrowing toenail

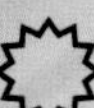

Incidence

This condition almost exclusively affects the hallux of teenagers and young adults.

Clinical features

It is caused by the sharp, distal edge of the toenail impinging on the adjacent nail fold. A superimposed infection causes redness, swelling, pain and intermittent discharge of pus (Figs 32, 33). The combination of acute inflammation and attempts at tissue repair result in the formation of exuberant granulation tissue around the laceration and surrounding inflammatory swelling.

Management

Conservative treatment

- Good hygiene – regular bathing, avoiding tight shoes, avoiding trauma
- 'Lift out' the ingrowing portion of the nail with a pledget of gauze or cotton wool

Surgical treatment

Operations are usually performed under local anaesthesia using a ring block and tourniquet.

- Removal of whole nail without disturbing the nail bed
- Wedge resection/phenolization for permanent narrowing of nail
- Zadek's operation for permanent ablation of nail bed

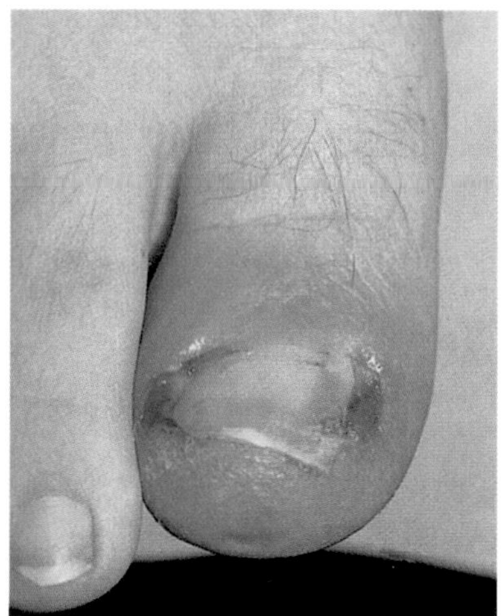

Fig. 32 Ingrowing toenail with super-added infection.

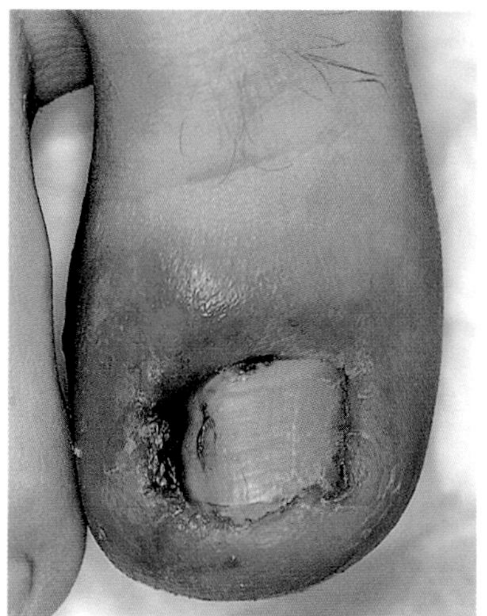

Fig. 33 Infected right ingrowing toenail.

Nail conditions

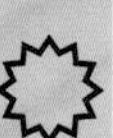

Onychogryphosis

This overgrowth of the nail resembles an ox or goat horn. One or more nails (most often the hallux) become grossly thickened, deformed and hypertrophic (Fig. 34).

Management

Avulsion of the nail does not prevent recurrence and excision of the nail with ablation of the nail bed is often required.

Nailfold infections (paronychia)

Clinical features

Pain, redness and swelling at the side and base of the nail are typical (Fig. 35). Extension under the nail and into the underlying pulp space may occur.

Management

- Antibiotics
- Surgical drainage

Finger clubbing

Definition

Initially the angle between the proximal nail fold and the nail is lost. The tissues beneath the nail and the finger pulp then become obviously swollen and finally the end of the finger swells laterally to produce a 'drumstick' appearance (Fig. 36).

Aetiology

There are many causes of finger clubbing, including congenital cyanotic heart disease, bronchial carcinoma, chronic chest sepsis, cirrhosis and inflammatory bowel disease.

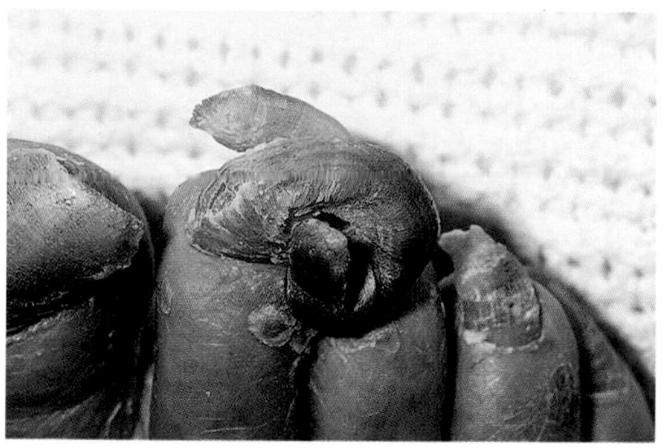

Fig. 34 Onychogryphosis.

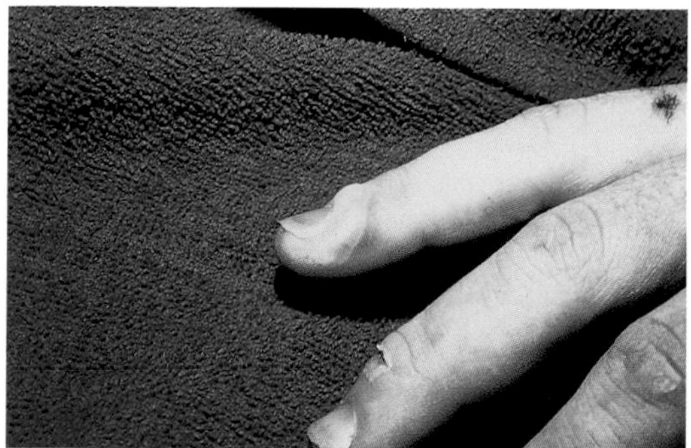

Fig. 35 Paronychia affecting the nail bed of the left index finger. This required surgical incision under digital block anaesthesia to release the pus.

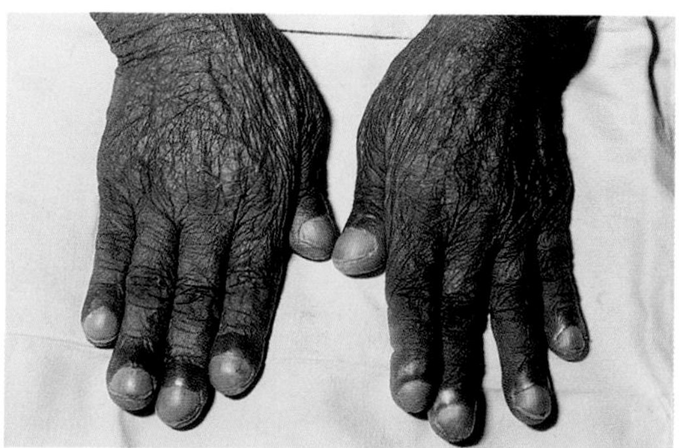

Fig. 36 Finger clubbing.

14 Branchial lesions

Branchial cyst

Incidence	Branchial cysts are uncommon. The cysts arise from remnants of the second pharyngeal pouch or brachial cleft. Although congenital, presentation is usually in late adolescence or early adulthood.
Clinical features	The patient typically complains of a painless swelling in the side of the neck that may vary in size from time to time. It is smooth, mobile and, unless infected, not tender.
Differential diagnosis	• Acute lymphadenitis • Tuberculosis
Management	Diagnosis can be confirmed by fine-needle aspiration, which reveals creamy material with cholesterol crystals on microscopy. Treatment is by surgical excision. Inflamed cysts may require urgent drainage.

Branchial fistula and sinus

Branchial fistulas or sinuses are even less common than branchial cysts and may be bilateral.

Clinical features	They present as a discharging opening near the lower end of the anterior border of the sternomastoid muscle (Fig. 37). A sinus ends blindly at the lateral pharyngeal wall whereas a fistula communicates with the oropharynx near the tonsillar fossa. Branchial fistulas are apparent soon after birth.
Management	Management is by surgical excision (Fig. 38).

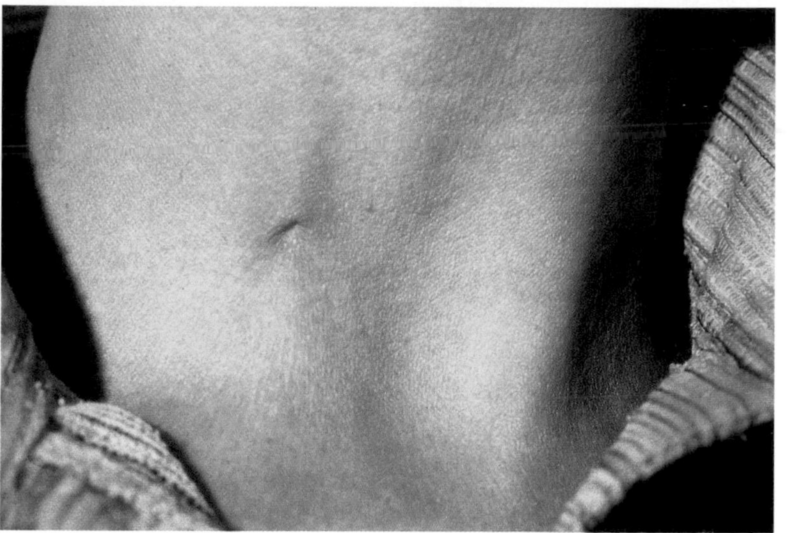

Fig. 37 Branchial fistula opening on to the neck that intermittently discharged mucus.

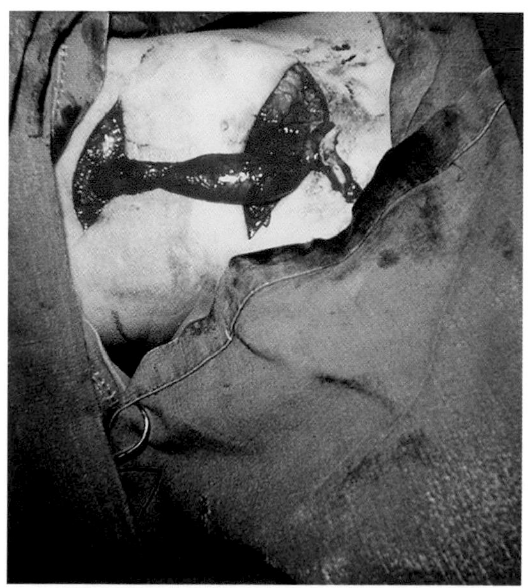

Fig. 38 Branchial fistula and cyst undergoing excision.

15 Lymphadenopathy in the head and neck

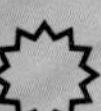

Classification

- Isolated lymphadenopathy (Fig. 39) – caused by local disease within its field of drainage, e.g. tonsillitis, dental infection
- Systemic lymphadenopathy – e.g. glandular fever, HIV
- Cervical tuberculosis – scrofula, cold abscess
- Lymphomas (Fig. 40)
- Secondary (metastatic) tumours – e.g. primaries in the head or neck, chest or abdomen (Fig. 41).

Clinical features

History

Important features are:

- Duration of the swelling
- Progression and size
- Associated pain
- Other symptoms, e.g. hoarseness, dysphagia
- Systemic symptoms, e.g. weight loss, night sweats.

Examination

Relevant information includes:

- Site and size
- Relationship to other anatomical structures
- Fixation to other structures
- Special features, e.g. pulsatile, presence of a bruit or thrill, tenderness, fluctuation.

Examination must include mouth, pharynx, nasopharynx, larynx and oesophagus.

Management

- Routine bloods, e.g. white cell count, Monospot
- Tumours from the chest or abdomen often metastasize to the lower part of the posterior triangle, particularly to Virchow's node, which lies deeply in the angle between the sternomastoid muscle and the clavicle on the left side
- Fine needle aspiration
- CT scanning – valuable when the likely diagnosis is metastatic nodal disease
- Chest X-ray – to exclude lung cancer, tuberculosis
- Complete excision of lymph node – may be required if fine needle aspiration is unhelpful.

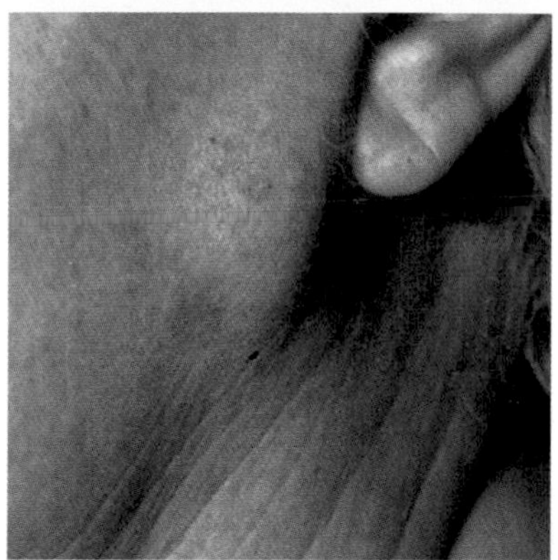

Fig. 39 A painless and hard jugulodigastric lymph node at the angle of the mandible.

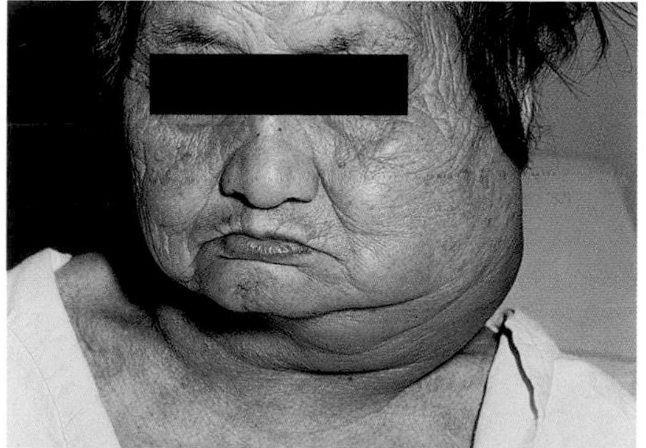

Fig. 40 Lymphadenopathy secondary to lymphoma.

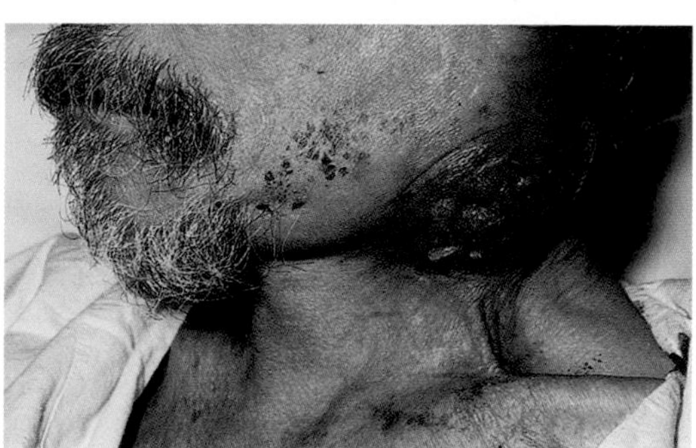

Fig. 41 Metastatic lymphadenopathy with erosion through the overlying skin due to spread from a primary squamous-cell carcinoma of the soft palate.

16 Non-neoplastic salivary gland disease

Classification

- Bacterial infection – parotitis, submandibular sialadenitis
- Viral parotitis
- Sialectasis

Parotitis

Clinical features

- The parotid gland swells, becomes acutely tender and the overlying skin may be slightly erythematous (Fig. 42)
- There may occasionally be a discharge of pus from the duct orifice, which lies above the second upper molar tooth

Management

Parotitis requires good mouth hygiene, rehydration and antibiotics. If fluctuation develops, incision and drainage of the abscess is necessary.

Sialectasis

This is most commonly seen in the submandibular gland. The swelling is often intermittent and painful, particularly after eating (Fig. 43A,B). The cause is often a single calculus at the duct orifice in the mouth. This may be palpable on bimanual examination. Alternatively a stone might be identified on an intraoral dental X-ray (Fig. 44).

Management

Intraoral incision of the duct and removal of the stone under local anaesthesia (Fig. 45). Widespread stone disease with destruction of glandular tissue leading to chronic inflammation requires excision of the entire gland. Damage to the lingual nerve must be avoided.

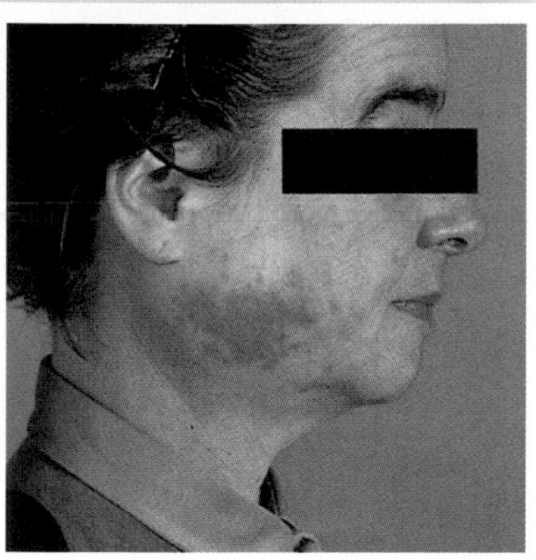

Fig. 42 Acute parotitis. This patient has a tender unilateral swelling in the region of the parotid gland. The overlying skin is stretched, shiny and reddened.

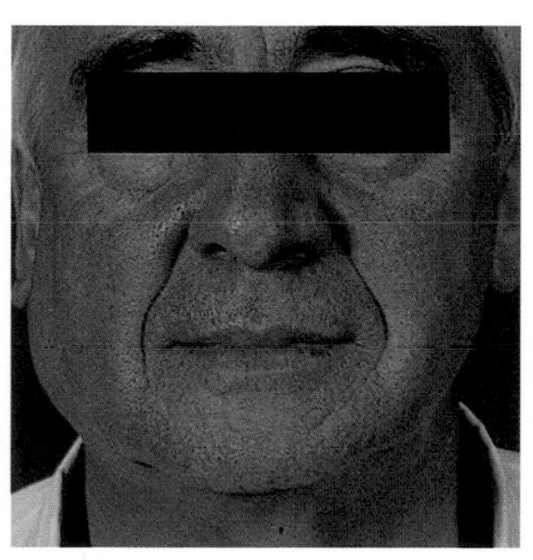

A

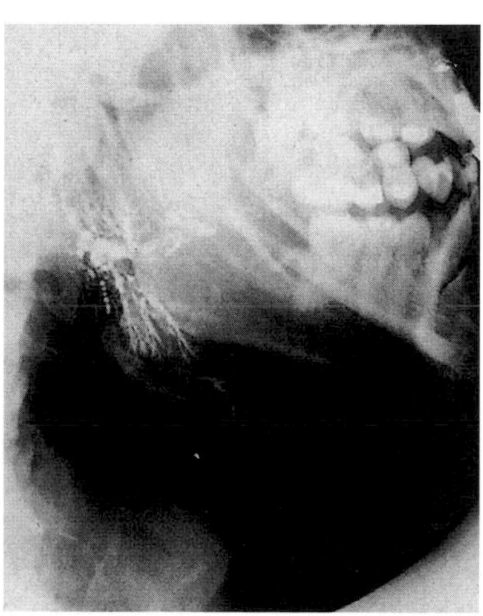

B

Fig. 43 A. Sialectasis affecting the right parotid gland. B. Sialography demonstrated a dilated duct system.

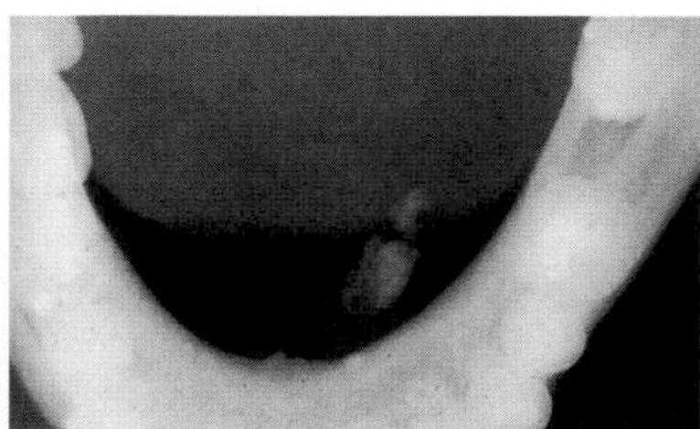

Fig. 44 Calculus obstructing the submandibular duct on plain X-ray which could be palpated on bimanual palpation.

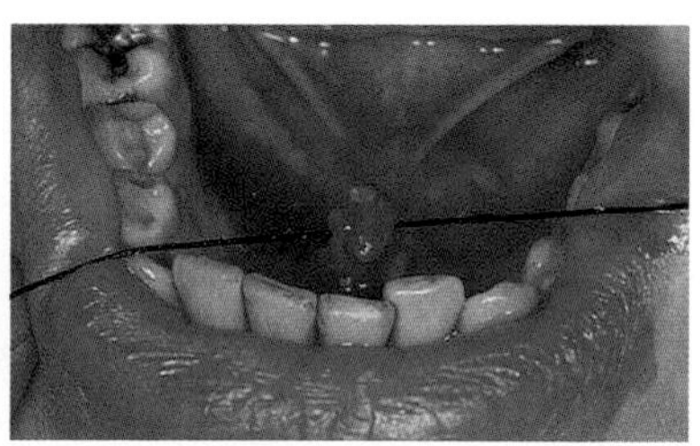

Fig. 45 The submandibular calculus was removed by opening the duct and extracting the calculus.

17 Parotid tumours

Classification

- Benign – pleomorphic adenoma, adenolymphoma
- Intermediate – oncocytoma, mucoepidermoid tumour
- Malignant – squamous carcinoma (Fig. 46)
- Adenocystic carcinoma, adenocarcinoma, lymphoma.

Most salivary gland tumours are benign. The smaller the gland the higher the chance of a tumour being malignant (70% of parotid tumours are benign, 70% of minor salivary gland tumours are malignant).

Clinical features

Pleomorphic adenoma presents as a painless mass, which may enlarge very slowly over a period of several years. The lump is usually discrete and mobile.

Benign tumours do not involve the facial nerve, in contrast to malignant tumours, which may present with a facial palsy (Fig. 47).

Management

Surgical excision is the definitive treatment. Pleomorphic adenomas have a capsule and rupture of this can lead to tumour seeding and recurrence. If a malignant parotid tumour is found to directly involve the facial nerve, this structure must be removed. A resected nerve can sometimes be successfully grafted.

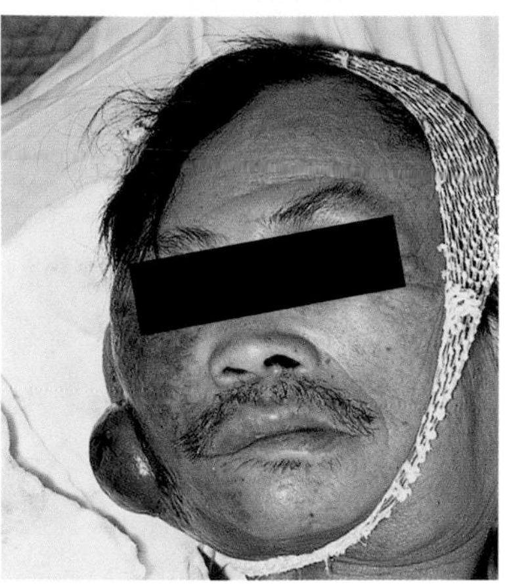

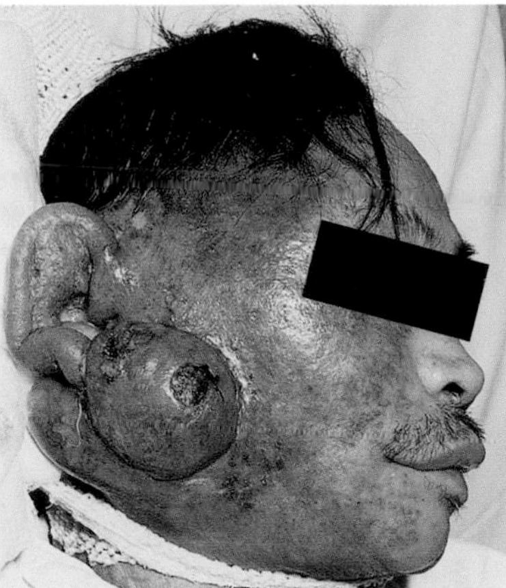

Fig. 46 A&B Advanced carcinoma of the left parotid gland.

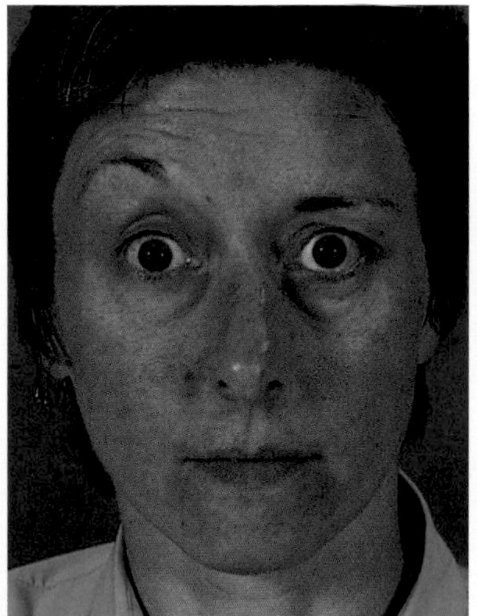

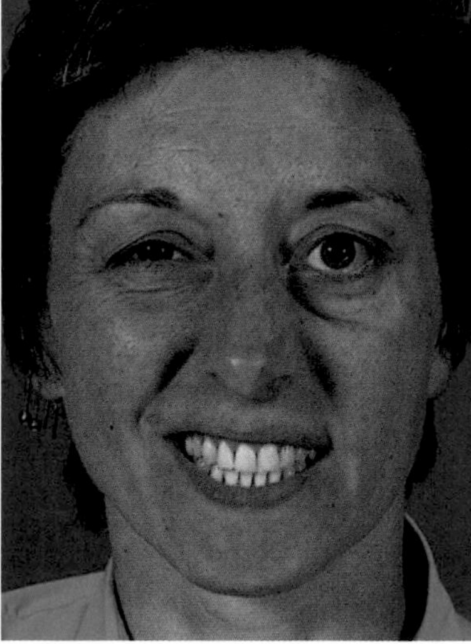

Fig. 47 A&B Partial facial nerve palsy following parotid surgery. Facial palsy can also be due to invasion of the facial nerve – uncommon but diagnostic of malignancy.

18 Thyroid gland

Thyroglossal cyst

Aetiology

The thyroid gland develops from the thyroglossal duct, which grows downwards from the area of the foramen caecum at the back of the tongue. The track usually disappears but islands of thyroid tissue may be deposited at any point along its course and develop into a thyroglossal cyst.

Clinical features

- Commonly presents during the second or third decade of life
- A midline swelling is visible that is separate from the thyroid gland itself (Figs 48, 49)
- The cyst moves upwards on protrusion of the tongue because it is attached to the base of the tongue.

Management

The thyroglossal cyst should be excised, together with the tract. To avoid recurrence, the central portion of the hyoid bone is included in the excision.

Thyroglossal fistula

Aetiology

This midline orifice can result from spontaneous discharge of an infected thyroglossal cyst. More commonly it follows excision or drainage of a cyst without removal of the tract.

Clinical features

The orifice discharges intermittently and may be associated with surrounding erythema and inflammation.

Management

Excision of the entire thyroglossal fistula tract.

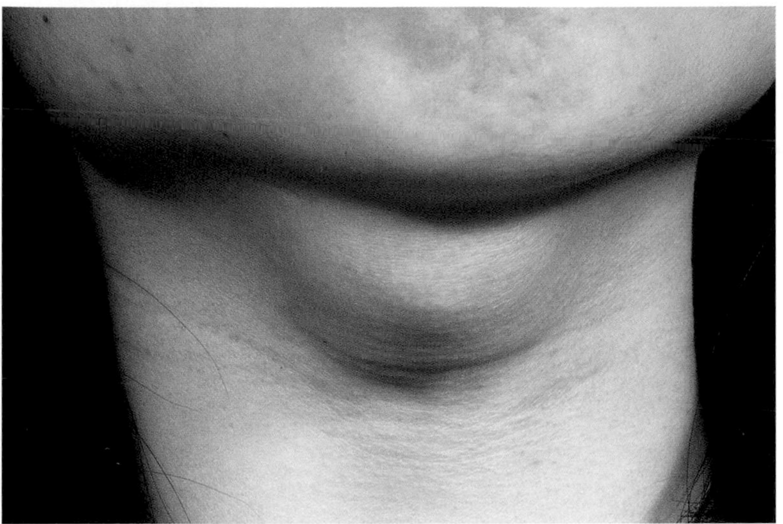

Fig. 48 Anterior view of thyroglossal cyst.

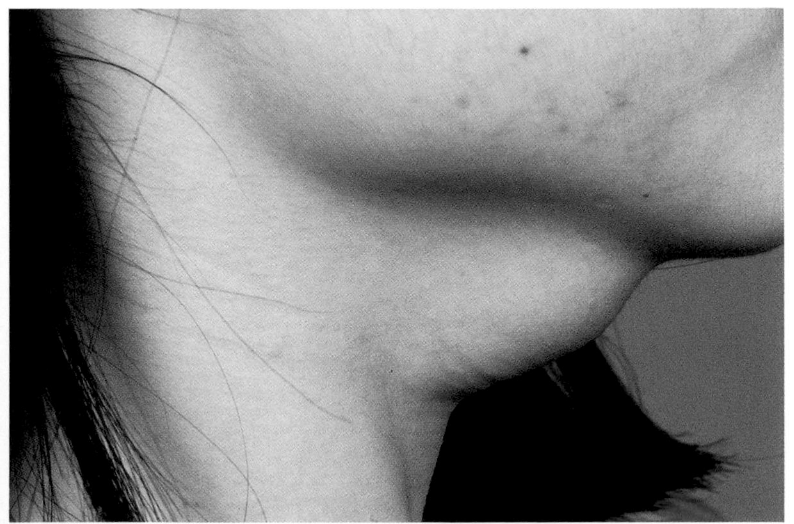

Fig. 49 Lateral view of thyroglossal cyst.

19 Thyroid goitre

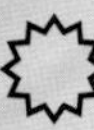

Classification

- Physiological enlargement, e.g. during puberty or pregnancy
- Non-toxic nodular goitre – endemic in some areas from iodine deficiency
- Thyrotoxic goitre
- Thyroiditis, e.g. De Quervain's disease, Hashimoto's disease, Riedel's thyroiditis
- Solitary thyroid nodules – 50% are part of a multinodular goitre, 25% are benign adenomas and 25% are cysts with differentiated cancers.

Clinical features

Symptoms may be related to a change in thyroid hormonal status and there may be associated neck symptoms such as:

- Dysphagia
- Dyspnoea
- Hoarse voice – implies infiltration of the recurrent laryngeal nerve

Characteristically there is swelling in the lower part of the neck that moves upwards on swallowing (Figs 50, 51). Swelling may be focal or diffuse. Occasionally a large goitre will descend behind the manubrium – this is detected by palpation in the suprasternal notch and percussion over the manubrium.

Investigation

- Thyroid function tests
- Ultrasound scan
- Radioisotope scan
- Fine needle aspiration cytology

Management

- Thyroid cysts can be aspirated and do not require excision
- Hyperfunctioning thyroid tissue should be removed by subtotal thyroidectomy (multinodular goitre) or lobectomy (toxic adenoma)
- Follicular neoplasms should be excised as differentiation between a follicular adenoma and follicular carcinoma cannot be determined by cytopathology
- Papillary carcinoma requires total thyroidectomy as the disease is commonly multifocal

Prognosis

- Papillary carcinoma has an excellent prognosis (10-year survival rate 90%)
- Follicular carcinoma is more aggressive (10-year survival rate 50%)
- Anaplastic carcinoma usually results in death within 6 months of diagnosis

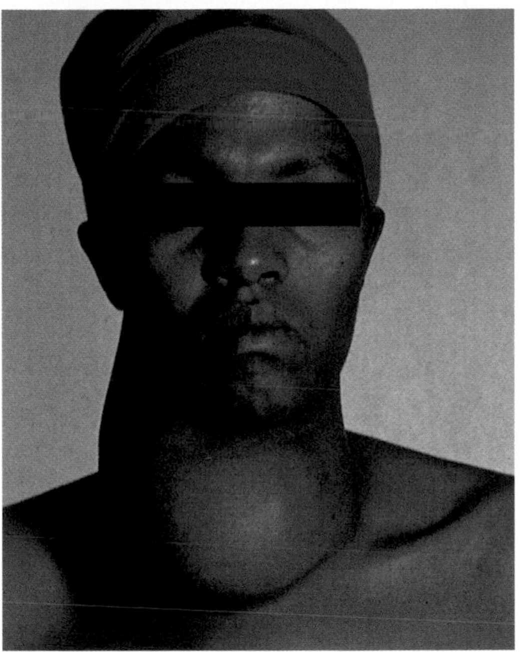

Fig. 50 Thyroid goitre in an asymptomatic patient.

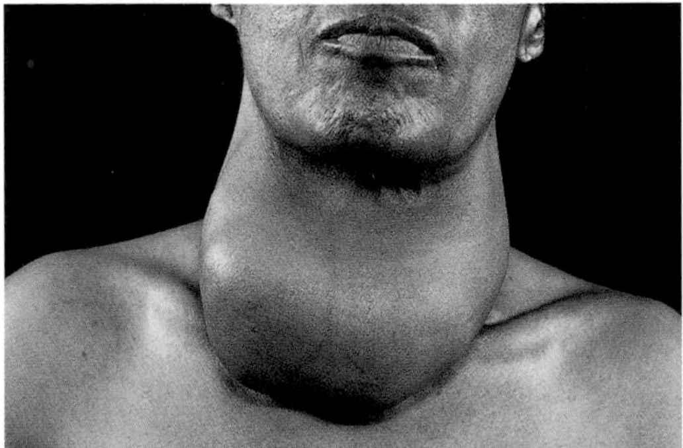

Fig. 51 Massive thyroid goitre.

20 Thyrotoxicosis/myxoedema

Thyrotoxicosis (hyperthyroidism)

Incidence

Thyrotoxicosis is a relatively common problem affecting nearly 2% of females and 0.5% of males.

Aetiology

- Diffuse toxic goitre – Graves disease (primary hyperthyroidism)
- Multinodular toxic goitre
- Toxic solitary nodule or adenoma.

Clinical features

The symptoms associated with hyperthyroidism include heat intolerance, irritability, weight loss, diarrhoea, muscle weakness, tremor, loss of libido and eye complaints. In Graves disease, the thyroid is uniformly enlarged, firm, smooth and may have a bruit on auscultation. The skin may be warm and sweaty. Pulse rate may be increased and atrial fibrillation is common. Eye changes may result in exophthalmos (protrusion of the eye; Figs 52, 53) and ophthalmoplegia due to retrobulbar fat deposition. The proptosis is extenuated by lid retraction. When asked to follow a finger slowly up and down, the upper lid lags.

Myxoedema (hypothyroidism)

Clinical features

The symptoms and signs of myxoedema are the reverse of thyrotoxicosis. Symptoms include cold intolerance, slowness, tiredness, malaise, weight gain, constipation and depression. The signs include:

- Hypersomnolence
- Slow relaxing tendon reflexes
- Nerve entrapment, e.g. carpal tunnel syndrome
- Cool, dry and thickened skin
- Coarse hair
- Peripheral and periorbital oedema
- Hoarse voice
- Bradycardia
- Cardiomegaly.

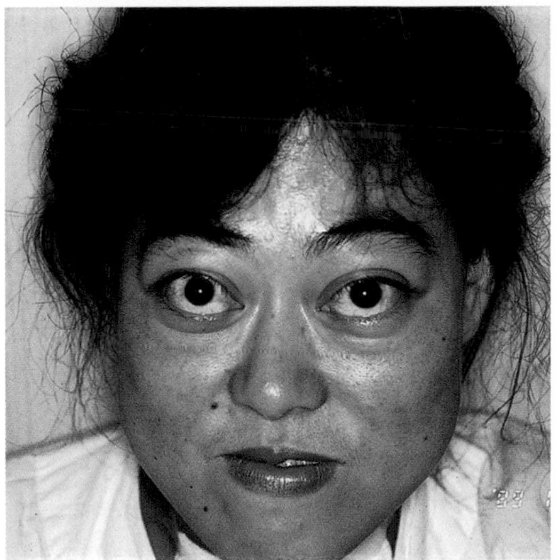

Fig. 52 A patient with thyrotoxicosis demonstrating exophthalmos.

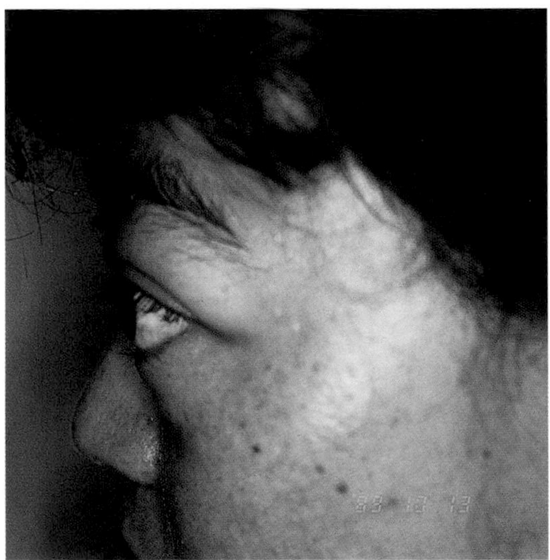

Fig. 53 Lateral view of same patient showing protrusion of the eye associated with thyrotoxicosis.

21 Benign breast disease

Clinical features

- Pain – cyclical or non-cyclical
- Solitary lump or lumpiness
- Nipple discharge
- Infection

Investigations

- Ultrasonography
- Mammography (Fig. 54)
- Magnetic resonance imaging
- Fine needle aspiration cytology
- Core biopsy (open biopsy)

Breast cyst

Incidence

Approximately 7% of women will develop a breast cyst at some time in their life. Cysts constitute approximately 15% of all discrete breast masses.

Clinical features

The history is of a palpable smooth discrete lump that can be painful. Physical findings are of a tense, discrete, mobile lump which is rarely fluctuant.

Management

Ultrasonography will reveal a well-demarcated hypoechoic lesion. Needle aspiration should be undertaken (Fig. 55). Cysts that refill or contain blood-stained fluid should be excised to exclude malignancy.

Fibroadenoma

Clinical features

Fibroadenoma commonly present in younger women as a solitary, discrete, mobile, non-tender lump – often referred to as a 'breast mouse'. A rare variant, usually in older women, is known as a phyllodes tumour.

Management

As with any discrete lump they should be subjected to triple assessment (clinical examination, imaging and fine needle aspiration cytology, FNAC). Small lesions do not require excision. Larger lesions (>4 cm) or those in older women should be considered for excision (Fig. 56).

Fibroadenosis

Clinical features

Fibroadenosis usually presents with a single lump or multiple lumps in the upper outer quadrant of the breast that are painful and tender premenstrually (i.e. cyclical).

Management

Provided that imaging (ultrasound or mammography) and FNAC have eliminated a malignancy, essentially the treatment is reassurance and medication for symptom relief.

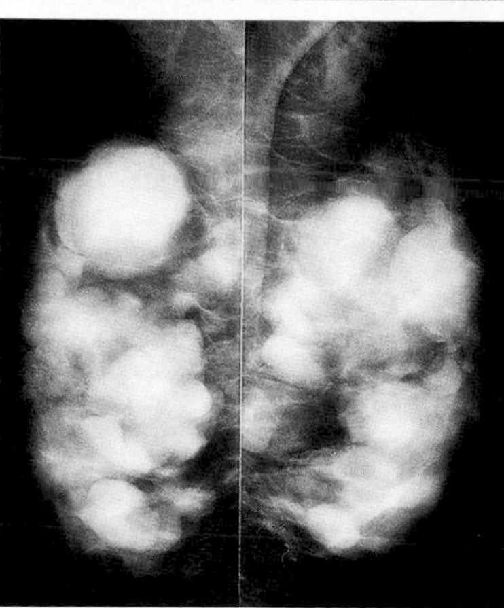

Fig. 54 Mammogram of multiple bilateral breast cysts.

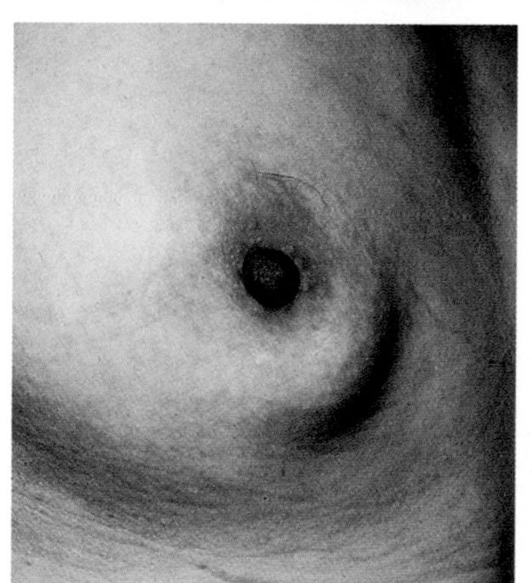

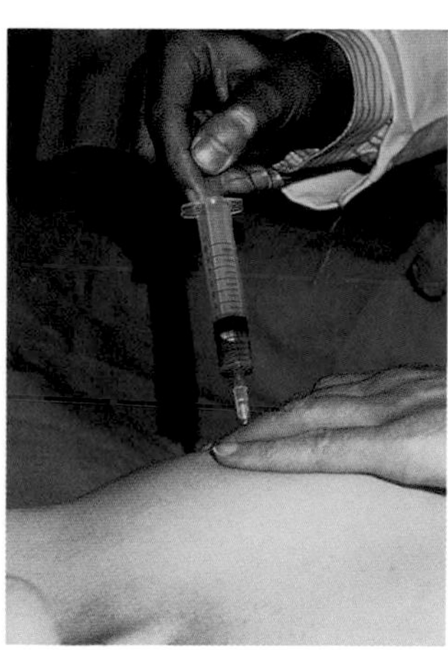

A B

Fig. 55 A. Palpable breast cyst. B. Aspiration of breast cyst.

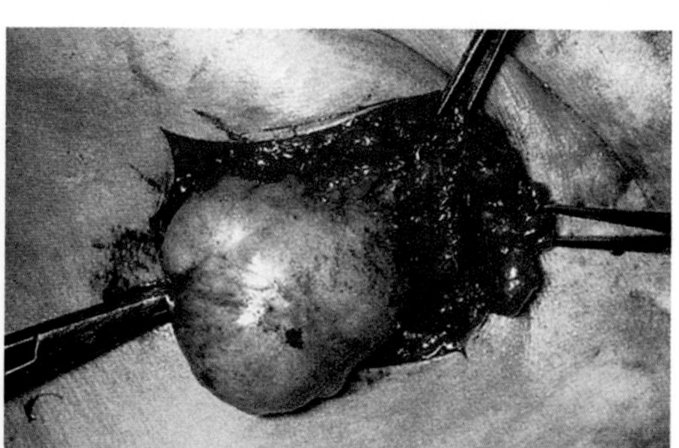

Fig. 56 Fibroadenoma being excised at open surgery.

22 Breast infection

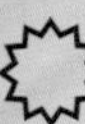

Incidence

Breast infection occurs occasionally in neonates but most commonly affects women aged between 18 and 50.

Classification

- Lactational breast abscess (Fig. 57) – the organism is most commonly *Staphylococcus aureus*
- Non-lactational breast abscess – anaerobes and aerobes are often responsible
- Periductal mastitis (Fig. 58) – characterized by a low-grade inflammatory response around the ducts adjacent to the nipple.

Clinical features

Diagnosis of breast infection is usually obvious, with local and systemic signs of acute inflammation. The affected segment of the breast is painful and tender, red and warm. If inadequately treated, an abscess forms and the lesion may eventually 'point' on the skin.

Management

The early cellulitic phase is reversible if treated with appropriate antibiotics. Continued pain suggests an underlying abscess which in its early stages can be treated with repeated aspiration and antibiotics. Skin changes such as necrosis or failure to settle with simple aspiration indicates formal incision and drainage under general anaesthetic.

Periductal mastitis

Incidence

This condition affects young women, predominantly in the fourth decade of life and is associated with smoking. It is characterized histologically by a low-grade inflammatory response around the ducts adjacent to the nipple. The bacteria involved are predominantly anaerobes.

Clinical features

Tenderness develops predominantly in one segment of the areola. A tender swelling at the edge of the areola may progress to abscess formation with a periareolar sinus and discharge (mamillary duct fistula; Fig. 59).

Management

FNAC and mammography may be necessary to exclude an underlying carcinoma. Inflammatory swellings may respond to antibiotics. If an abscess develops it requires the same treatment as a lactational abscess, which is usually drainage rather than aspiration. If a mammary duct fistula develops it requires excision of the duct segment.

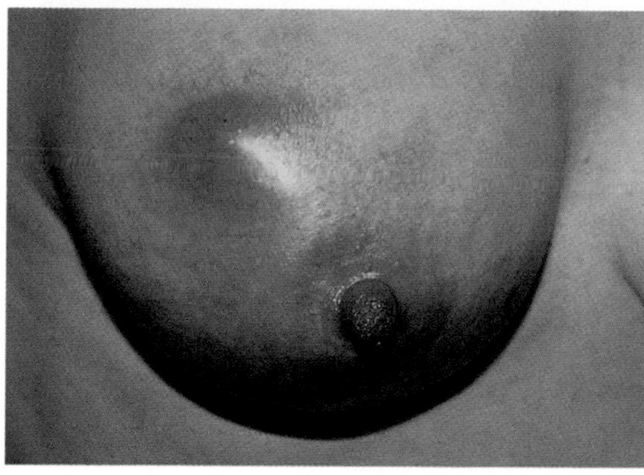

Fig. 57 Lactational breast abscess. These usually occur within the first few weeks of breast feeding and are characteristically due to *Staphylococcus aureus*.

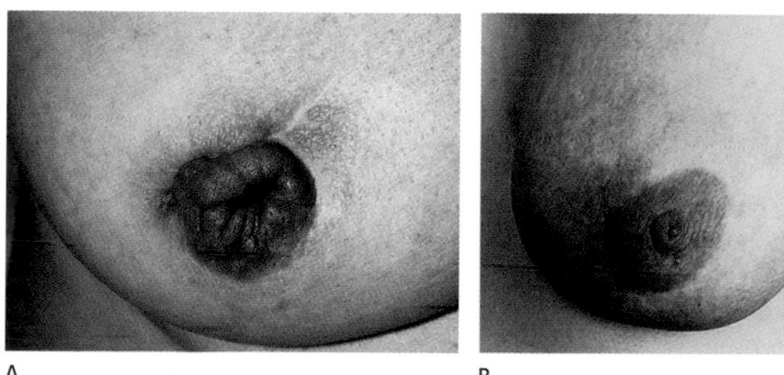

A B

Fig. 58 A. Nipple inversion due to periductal mastitis. **B.** Periductal mastitis.

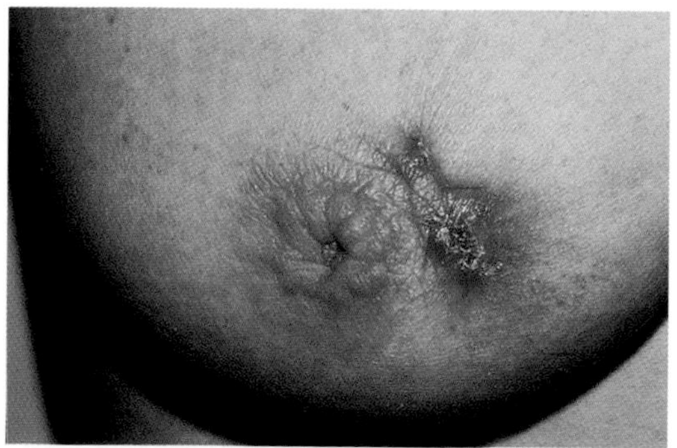

Fig. 59 Mammary duct fistula.

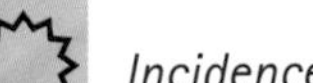

23 Abnormal breast tissue

Accessory nipple/breast tissue

Incidence

Between 1% and 4% of women have an accessory nipple (Fig. 60). The development of an accessory breast is unusual but they may even lactate if fully formed.

Clinical features

The presence of one or more vestigial nipples occur in the milk-line, which runs from the axilla down the anterior chest and abdomen and into the groin. The most common position for an accessory nipple is below the breast and above the umbilicus. The most common site for accessory breast tissue is in the axilla.

Management

Reassurance, but if the lesion is cosmetically unacceptable it can be excised under local anaesthesia.

Gynaecomastia

Incidence

Gynaecomastia (the growth of breast tissue in males) is entirely benign and usually reversible. It commonly occurs at puberty and 30–60% of boys aged 10–16 years have benign hypertrophy of the breast disc (Fig. 61). Senescent gynaecomastia usually affects men between 50 and 80 years of age. It is usually caused by drugs, liver cirrhosis, hypogonadism and, rarely, testicular tumours.

Management

Pubertal gynaecomastia requires no treatment as 80% resolves spontaneously within 2 years. A diagnosis of breast cancer should be excluded. Surgery may be indicated if the lesion is cosmetically unacceptable.

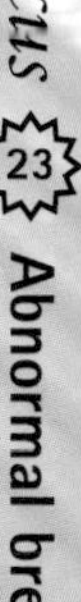

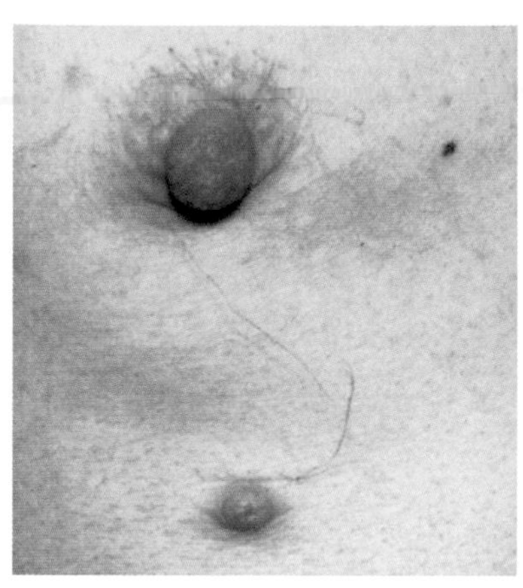

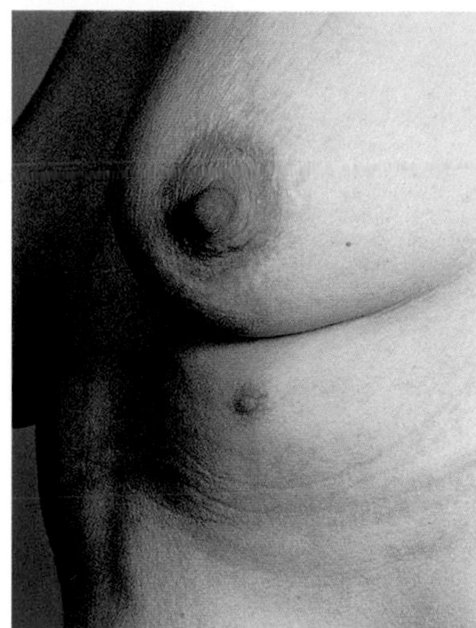

Fig. 60 A&B Accessory nipple.

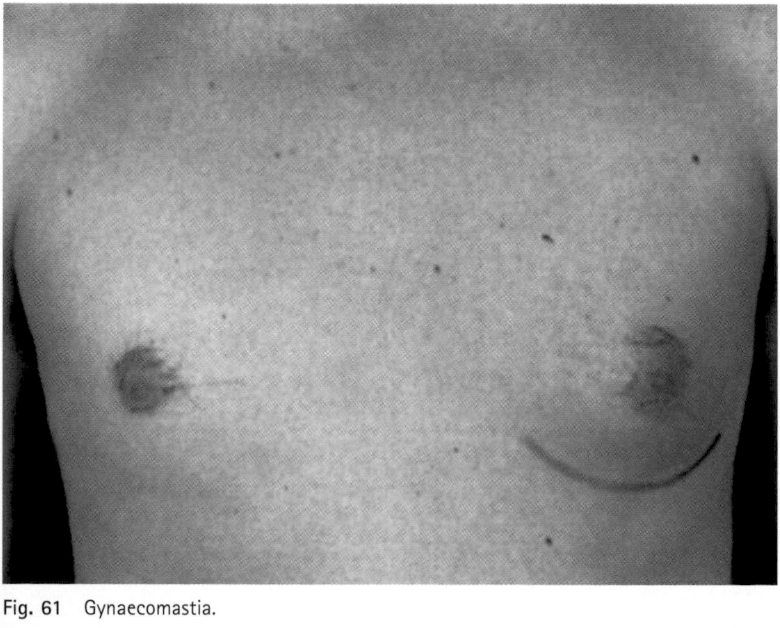

Fig. 61 Gynaecomastia.

24 Nipple abnormalities

Nipple discharge

There are three common causes:

- Mammary duct ectasia
- Duct papilloma
- Galactorrhoea.

Clinical features

It is important to establish whether the discharge is from a single or from multiple ducts. That from a single duct, particularly if blood stained, is more likely to be associated with a papilloma (Fig. 62). Careful examination of the breast is required to exclude a carcinoma. All nipple discharges should be sent for cytology which will frequently help with the diagnosis.

Management

Provided that imaging and cytological assessment indicate a diagnosis of mammary duct ectasia, reassurance may be all that is required. However, if a discharge is very troublesome, excision of the duct system (Hadfield's operation) provides symptomatic relief. If a duct papilloma is suspected the involved duct system should be excised.

Nipple retraction

Initially this may occur at puberty when the nipple is tethered as the breast grows. It is vital therefore to ask the patient if the retraction is long-standing or a recent change. Nipple retraction in later life (Fig. 63) is most often due to fibroadenosis but can be a sign of malignancy. If associated with a lump then further radiological imaging and FNAC is required.

Paget's disease

This is an eczematous condition of the nipple/areola complex (Fig. 64). It should be differentiated from eczema of the nipple. Paget's disease always involves the nipple and only involves the areola as a secondary event, whereas eczema primarily involves the areola and only secondarily affects the nipple. It is assumed that an underlying carcinoma is always present and treatment is by mastectomy.

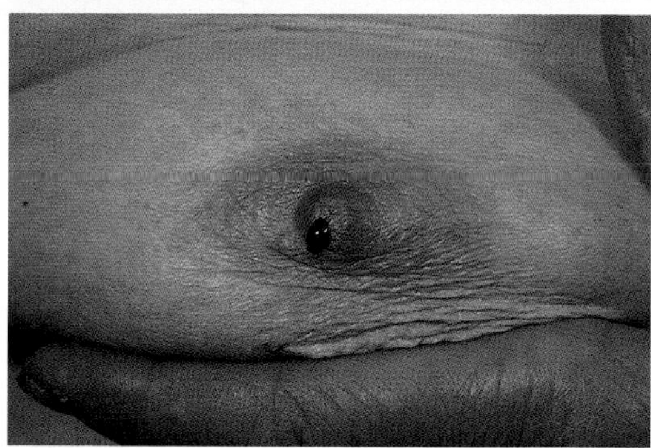

Fig. 62 Blood-stained nipple discharge from a single duct due to a duct papilloma.

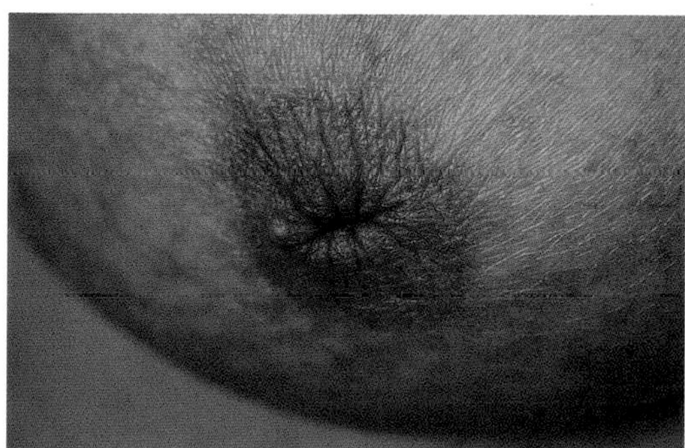

Fig. 63 Nipple retraction due to duct ectasia.

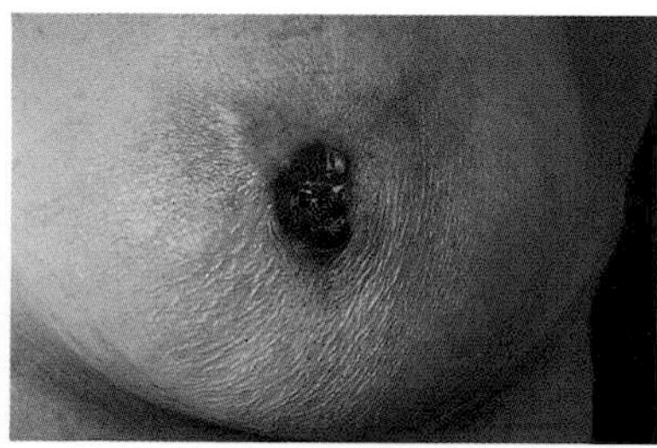

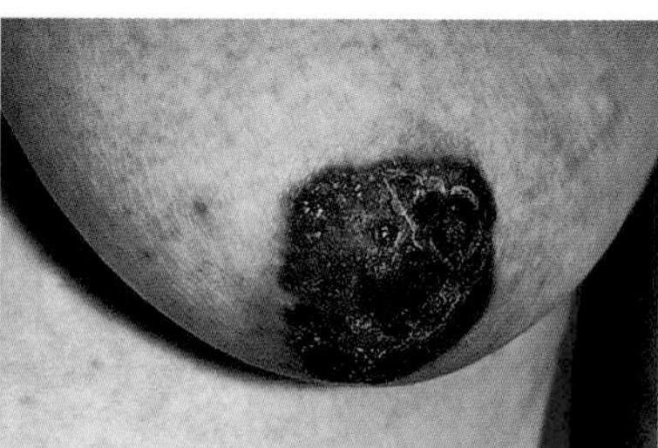

Fig. 64 A&B Paget's disease of the nipple.

25 Breast cancer

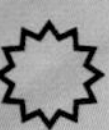

Incidence

Approximately 1 million new cases of breast cancer are diagnosed each year worldwide. It is the commonest malignancy in women and comprises 18% of all female cancers. In the UK, approximately 1 in 10 women will develop breast cancer. Risk factors for breast cancer are:

- Increasing age
- Increased age at first pregnancy
- Nulliparity
- Previous history of benign breast disease
- Family history.

Clinical features

The most common presentation is with a breast lump, which is usually painless. Other symptoms may include nipple retraction (4%), nipple discharge (2%), skin retraction (1%) or an axillary mass (1%).

Malignant lesions are usually firm and irregular and often produce visible signs of breast asymmetry, such as dimpling/puckering of the overlying skin (Fig. 65), or retraction/alteration in nipple contour. With locally advanced disease, the lymphatic channels are obstructed and the skin becomes oedematous and thickened with prominent hair follicles (peau d'orange; Fig. 66).

Investigations

Any palpable breast abnormality should be assessed by the process of triple assessment:

- Clinical evaluation
- Radiological evaluation (Fig. 67)
- Cytological/histological evaluation.

Management

The principles of management of breast cancer are to:

- Control the disease in the affected breast and chest wall
- Treat local and regional disease in early breast cancer
- Control advanced and disseminated disease (Fig. 68).

Conservative surgery is the favoured approach. Mastectomy is indicated in patients with multifocal tumours or extensive non-invasive disease, those with previous incomplete excision or some women with large central tumours. If an axillary node clearance is performed, radiotherapy for positive nodes is unnecessary. Chemotherapy or hormonal therapy may be given as an adjuvant therapy after surgery and/or radiotherapy, as primary therapy or as neoadjuvant therapy before surgery and/or radiotherapy.

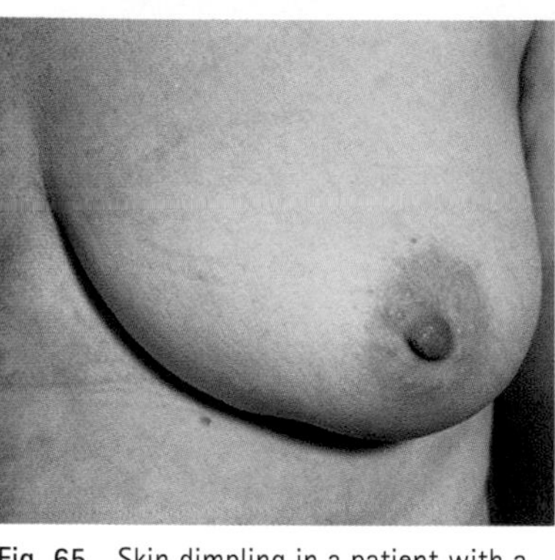

Fig. 65 Skin dimpling in a patient with a left breast carcinoma.

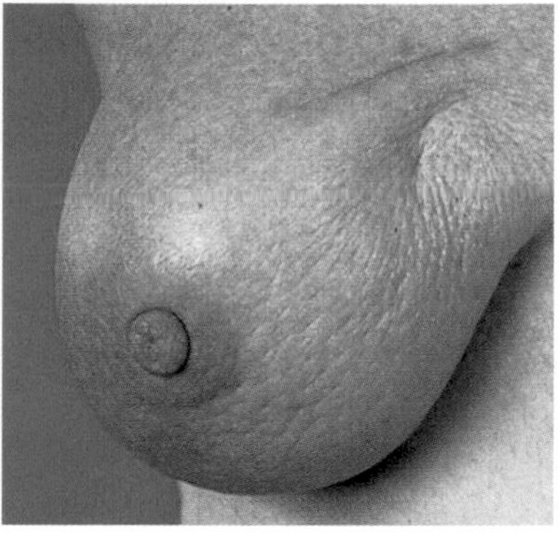

Fig. 66 Peau d'orange is a sign of locally advanced breast cancer.

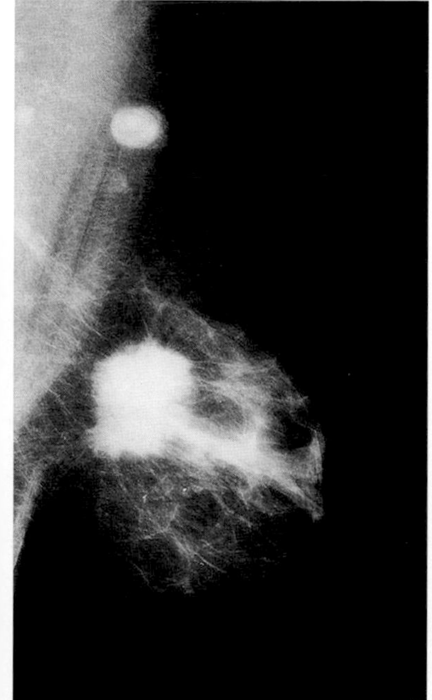

Fig. 67 Mammogram of breast carcinoma with an enlarged pathological axillary lymph node.

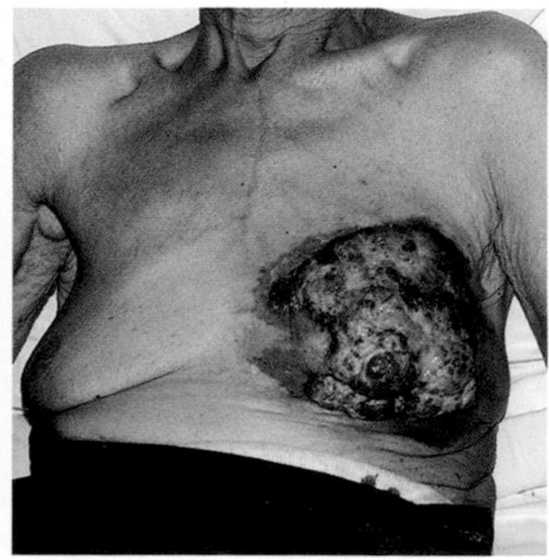

Fig. 68 Advanced carcinoma of the breast.

26 Jaundice

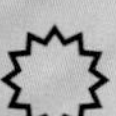

Definition

A yellowish discoloration of body tissues, due to an increase in serum bilirubin concentration. It usually becomes clinically apparent when levels exceed 35 µmol/l.

Classification

- Prehepatic – due to haemolysis
- Hepatic (or hepatocellular) – due to dysfunction of hepatocytes, e.g. viral hepatitis, hepatotoxic drugs, Gilbert's disease
- Posthepatic (or obstructive jaundice) – causes include obstruction in the lumen of the biliary tree (e.g. gallstones), obstruction in the wall of the bile ducts (e.g. cholangiocarcinoma, postoperative stricture) or extrinsic compression (e.g. pancreatic cancer, porta hepatis nodes, pancreatitis; Fig. 69).

Clinical features

Important aspects of the history are to ascertain occupation, social habits, drug and alcohol history, information about overseas travel and previous blood transfusions. A history of intermittent pain, fluctuant jaundice and dyspepsia suggests choledocholithiasis whereas a history of weight loss and progressive jaundice favours a diagnosis of malignancy. Obstructive jaundice is likely if there is a history of dark urine, pale stools and itch. Hepatocellular jaundice is likely if there are stigmata of chronic liver disease, such as palmar erythema, spider naevi and gynaecomastia. The abdomen must be examined for evidence of hepatomegaly or gallbladder distension and for signs of portal hypertension, such as splenomegaly, ascites and large collateral veins (caput medusae). Courvoisier's law states that obstructive jaundice in the presence of a palpable gall bladder is not due to gallstones and is therefore likely to be caused by a tumour.

Investigations

- Liver function tests
- Coagulation screen
- Hepatitis screen
- Full blood count – anaemia may signify haemolysis
- Ultrasonography (Fig. 70)
- CT scan – this may identify tumours and metastases
- Magnetic resonance cholangiopancreatography (MRCP)
- Endoscopic retrograde cholangiopancreatography (ERCP)
- Percutaneous transhepatic cholangiography (PTC)
- Laparoscopic staging
- Liver biopsy – can be performed percutaneously, during laparoscopy or by employing a transjugular approach

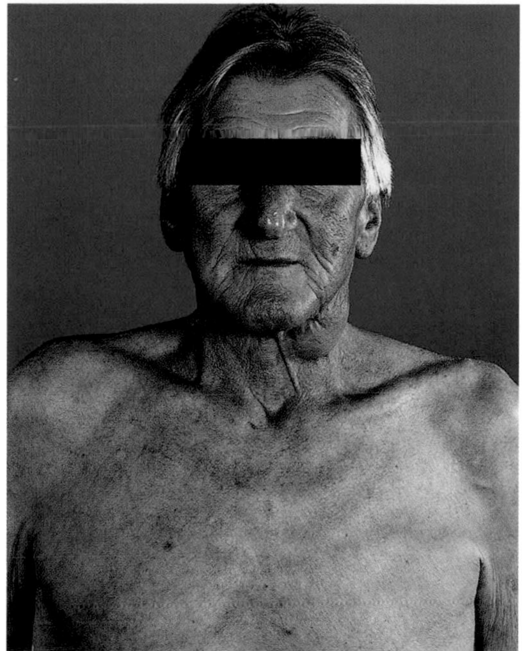

Fig. 69 Patient with jaundice due to malignant obstruction of the extrahepatic biliary tree secondary to pancreatic carcinoma.

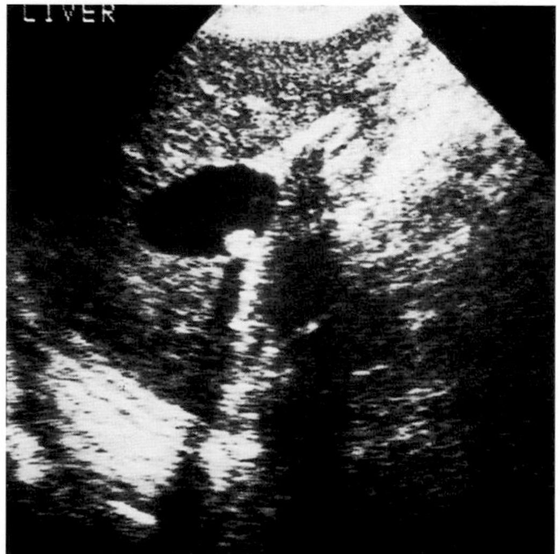

Fig. 70 Ultrasound scan demonstrating a gallstone within the gallbladder with posterior acoustic shadowing.

27 Gallstones

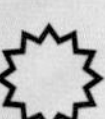

Incidence

Gallstones (Figs 71–73) are very common, with a prevalence of 10%. Incidence increases with age. They are two to four times more common in women and the typical patient is a 'fair, fat, fertile female in her fifties'.

Aetiology

Gallstones are formed from the constituents of bile and can be cholesterol stones, pigment stones or mixed stones. Predisposing factors to gallstone formation are:

- Cholesterol super-saturation
- Bile stasis
- Increased bilirubin secretion.

Clinical features

Gallstones may remain asymptomatic (silent) and therefore undetected for many years. Gallstones usually become clinically evident by the complications they cause, including:

- Biliary colic – constant pain, which can last from a few minutes to several hours
- Acute cholecystitis – tenderness and guarding are usually present in the right upper quadrant; there is often associated pyrexia
- Empyema – formation of pus within the gallbladder
- Mucocele – a distended gallbladder full of clear mucus
- Chronic cholecystitis – chronic inflammation of the gallbladder
- Obstructive jaundice – due to choledocholithiasis (gallstones in the bile duct)
- Cholangitis – characterized by abdominal pain, high fever with rigors and jaundice (sometimes termed Charcot's triad)
- Pancreatitis
- Gallstone ileus – a large gallstone erodes from gallbladder into small intestine and then impacts, usually in the terminal ileum

Management

Asymptomatic gallstones require no treatment. Cholecystectomy is indicated for symptomatic gallstones. Elderly patients with significant comorbidity presenting with acute cholecystitis or empyema, should undergo cholecystostomy (drainage of the gallbladder) which can be performed percutaneously under radiological guidance. Patients with acute cholangitis require systemic antibiotics and urgent relief of biliary obstruction.

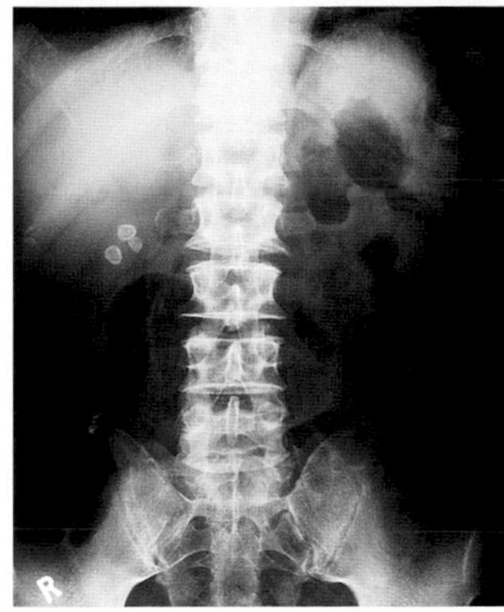

Fig. 71 Plain abdominal X-ray showing gallstones in the right upper quadrant.

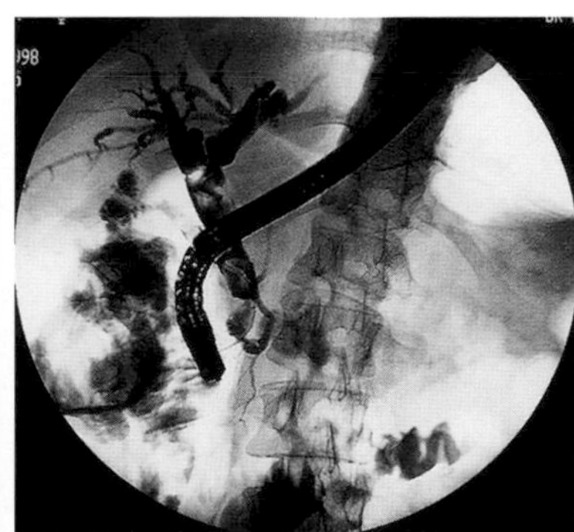

Fig. 72 ERCP demonstrating multiple calculi in the extrahepatic biliary tree.

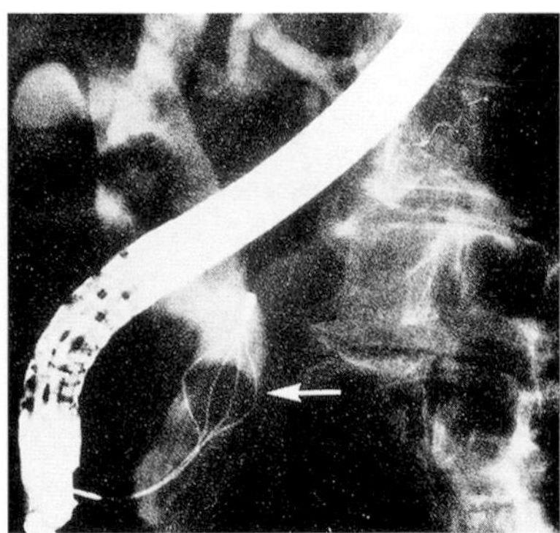

Fig. 73 ERCP showing basket extraction of ductal calculi.

28 Intestinal obstruction

Aetiology

- Small bowel – adhesions, hernias
- Large bowel – carcinoma, diverticular disease.

Clinical features

The four cardinal symptoms are:

- Abdominal pain
- Vomiting
- Abdominal distension
- Absolute constipation – for both faeces and flatus.

Features suggesting strangulation of the bowel include localized pain, tachycardia, pyrexia and peritonism.

Small bowel obstruction Vomiting occurs early and may lead to dehydration. Visible peristalsis may be seen. An abdominal scar suggests adhesions as a potential cause. An irreducible mass at a hernial orifice may indicate the aetiology. Increased bowel sounds that are high-pitched and tinkling are a classical sign.

Large bowel obstruction Gross distension may occur. While constipation occurs early, vomiting may be a later feature. Rectal examination may reveal an obstructing tumour.

Differential diagnosis

- Ascites
- Gross faecal loading
- Pregnancy
- Functional obstruction (pseudo-obstruction)

Investigations

- Plain abdominal X-rays – the characteristic appearance of small bowel obstruction is of distended loops of bowel with visible valvulae conniventes (Fig. 74). Large bowel obstruction may be demonstrated as peripheral distended bowel with visible haustrations (Fig. 75).
- Contrast X-rays. If large bowel obstruction is suspected, a retrograde contrast study should be performed (Fig. 76).
- CT scan – may elucidate cause.

Management

The indications for conservative management are:

- No evidence of strangulation or perforation
- Incomplete adhesive small bowel obstruction that can be managed by nasogastric intubation and intravenous fluids

Operative intervention is indicated for:

- Suspected strangulation, including those patients with irreducible hernias
- Complete large bowel obstruction with tenderness in the right iliac fossa indicating a closed loop obstruction
- Failure of resolution after a period of conservative management.

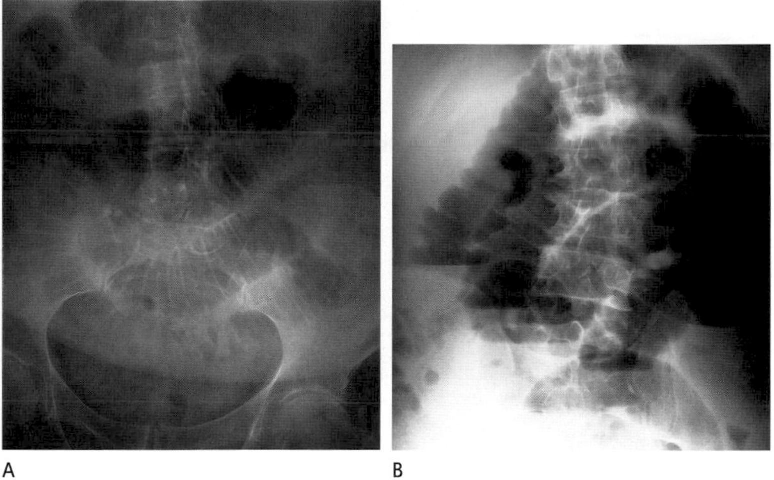

A B

Fig. 74 (A) Supine abdominal x-ray showing evidence of small bowel obstruction. Note the valvulae conniventes which pass across the entire width of the bile lumen. (B) Erect abdominal x-ray showing evidence of small bowel obstruction. Note the fluid levels.

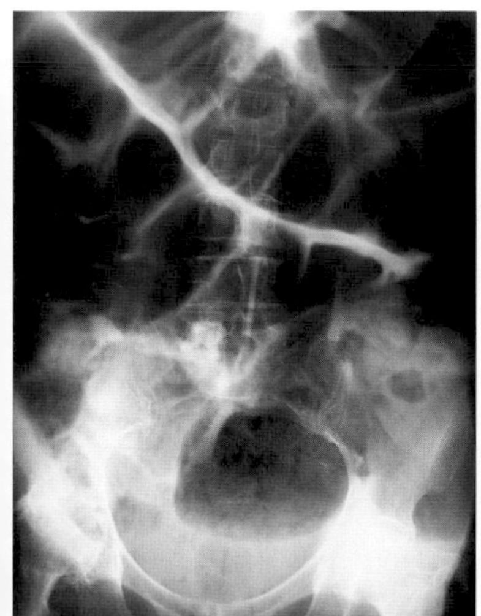

Fig. 75 Large bowel obstruction on abdominal x-ray. Note the haustrations which are the markings partially across the bowel lumen.

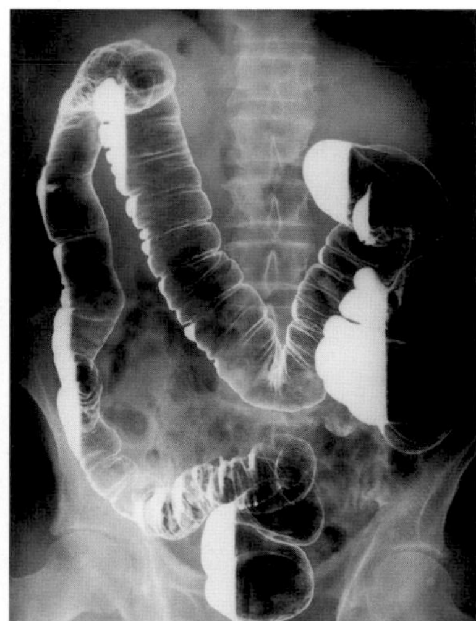

Fig. 76 Barium enema demonstrating a classical 'apple core' lesion of the descending colon.

29 Ascites

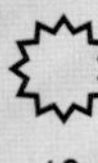

Definition

Ascites is defined as an accumulation of free fluid within the peritoneal cavity and has many causes, both malignant and non-malignant.

Aetiology

- Chronic liver disease
- Portal vein obstruction
- Hepatic vein obstruction
- Liver malignancy
- Hypoalbuminaemia – nephrotic syndrome, malnutrition
- Raised central venous pressure – congestive cardiac failure
- Malignancy
- Chylous ascites
- Pancreatic ascites
- Inflammatory disease.

Clinical features

Ascites results in abdominal distension (Figs 77, 78). It is characterized by dullness to percussion in the flanks when the patient is lying supine. 'Shifting dullness' may be demonstrated if the patient lies on one side resulting in alteration of the level in which resonance on percussion gives way to dullness owing to fluid gravitating to the dependent part of the peritoneal cavity. A 'fluid thrill' may also be elicited in patients with ascites.

Investigations

Ascites produces a ground-glass appearance on plain abdominal X-ray. Ultrasonography can detect as little as 50 ml of free fluid and may be used to confirm the diagnosis. Paracentesis performed under local anaesthesia can be used to relieve discomfort and obtain samples of ascitic fluid for bacteriology, cytology and biochemistry (Fig. 79).

Management

Management is directed at the cause of ascites where possible. Bed rest, restriction of sodium intake (and in some cases water intake) and diuretic therapy are the mainstays of treatment of non-malignant ascites. Intractable ascites may be an indication for peritovenous shunting or a transjugular intrahepatic portosystemic shunt (TIPSS) procedure. The installation of chemotherapeutic drugs (e.g. bleomycin) may be considered for malignant symptomatic ascites.

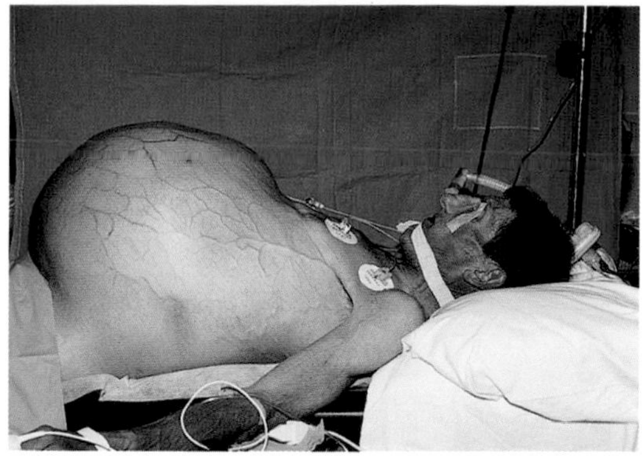

Fig. 77 Patient with significant ascites due to pseudomyxoma peritonei.

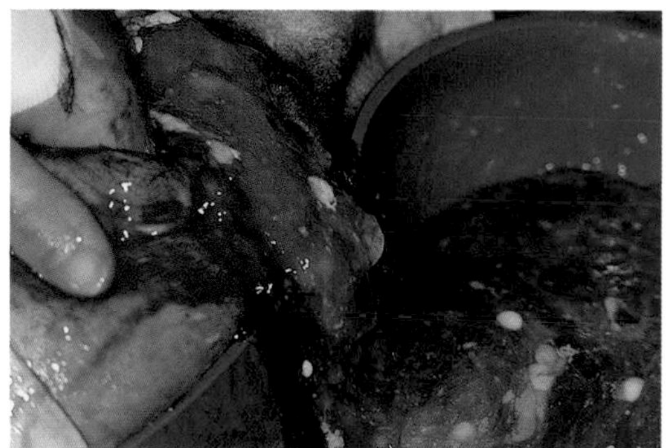

Fig. 78 Mucinous material removed at laparotomy from above patient.

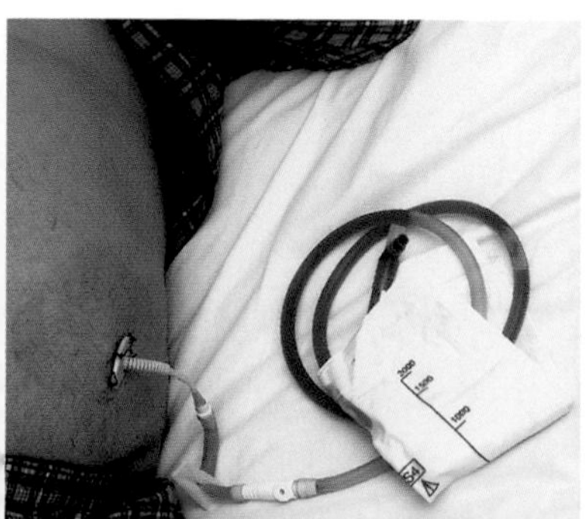

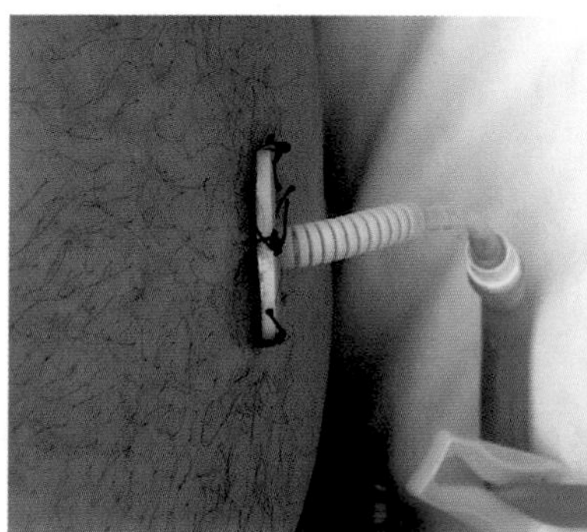

Fig. 79 A&B Paracentesis drain in left iliac fossa.

30 Acute pancreatitis

Incidence

In the UK approximately 100–200 per million of the population develop acute pancreatitis per annum.

Aetiology

- Gallstones
- Alcohol
- Viral infections, e.g. mumps, Coxsackie
- Drugs, e.g. steroids
- Hyperparathyroidism – hypercalcaemia
- Hyperlipidaemia
- Hypothermia
- Pancreatic cancer
- Post ERCP – 2–6% incidence
- Blunt or penetrating trauma

Clinical features

Abdominal pain radiating through to the back is usually prominent. Nausea and vomiting are often early features. The patient is usually restless but the pain may be relieved by leaning forward.

Examination may reveal upper abdominal tenderness. Shock is often present in severe pancreatitis. Bruising around the umbilicus (Cullen's sign) or brawny discoloration of the flanks (Gray Turner's sign; Fig. 80) are uncommon, relatively late signs of severe acute pancreatitis, but are indicative of a poor prognosis.

Investigations

- Serum amylase
- Liver function tests – may implicate a gallstone aetiology
- Scoring systems may predict the severity of an attack, e.g. Glasgow criteria, Ranson criteria, APACHE score
- Ultrasound scan – to look for gallstones
- Chest X-ray – pleural effusion is seen in 20% of cases
- CT scan – may reveal pancreatic necrosis in patients with severe acute pancreatitis (Fig. 81)

Management

Mild attacks are managed by fluid resuscitation and analgesia. Subsequent management is aimed at treating predisposing factors – cholecystectomy for gallstones.

Initial management of severe pancreatitis is supportive to maintain adequate organ function. Selective use of antibiotics may be beneficial, although this remains controversial. ERCP with sphincterotomy is recommended for patients with associated cholangitis. Enteral feeding may decrease morbidity. Pancreatic necrosectomy may be required.

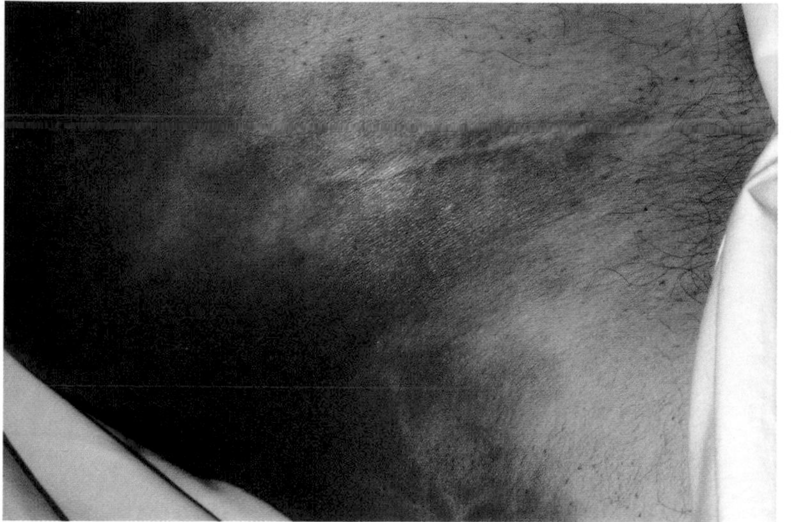

Fig. 80 Gray Turner's sign in a patient with severe acute pancreatitis.

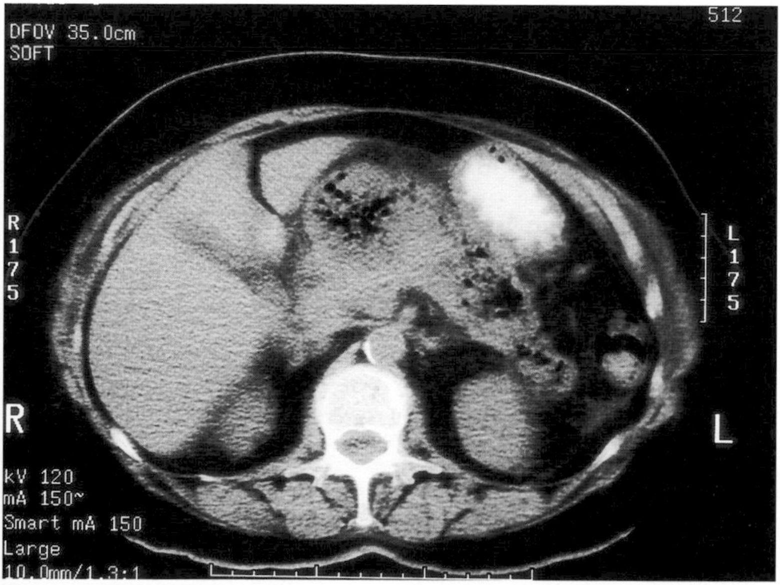

Fig. 81 CT scan demonstrating acute fluid collection and gas associated with severe acute pancreatitis.

31 Chronic pancreatitis

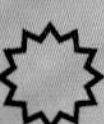

Definition

Chronic pancreatitis is a chronic inflammatory condition characterized by permanent structural or functional abnormality.

Clinical features

Pain is the principle symptom. It is characteristically epigastric with radiation to the back and is often eased by leaning forward. The application of heat sometimes brings relief but may result in permanent discoloration of the skin (erythema ab igne; Fig. 82). The progressive use of powerful opioid analgesics can result in drug dependency. Weight loss is usual and reflects a combination of inadequate intake, poor diet and malabsorption. Steatorrhoea is common; the bowel motion being pale, bulky, offensive, floats on water and is difficult to flush. Diabetes mellitus develops in about one-third of patients. Other less common manifestations of chronic pancreatitis included transient or intermittent obstructive jaundice, duodenal obstruction, portal vein thrombosis and pseudocyst formation.

Investigations

Abdominal plain films and CT scans may demonstrate speckled calcification typical of chronic pancreatitis (Fig. 83). They may also reveal pseudocysts, dilatation of the pancreatic duct and splenomegaly. MRCP or ERCP may delineate an abnormal or distorted pancreatic ductal system, which may contain pancreatic calculi.

Pancreatic endocrine function is assessed by random measurement of blood glucose levels. Exocrine function can be assessed by measuring faecal fat excretion but this is rarely undertaken in routine clinical practice.

Management

Conservative management consists of encouraging abstinence from alcohol, relief of pain, treatment of exocrine and endocrine insufficiency and attempts to improve nutritional status. Surgery is indicted if pain cannot be controlled by conservative means or if complications ensue. If the pancreatic duct system is distended, pancreaticojejunostomy is the operation of choice. If the duct system is not distended, partial or even total pancreatectomy may be necessary. Pancreatic pseudocysts can be drained endoscopically, laparoscopically or at open surgery. It is optimal to obtain dependent drainage either into the stomach or into a limb of jejunum.

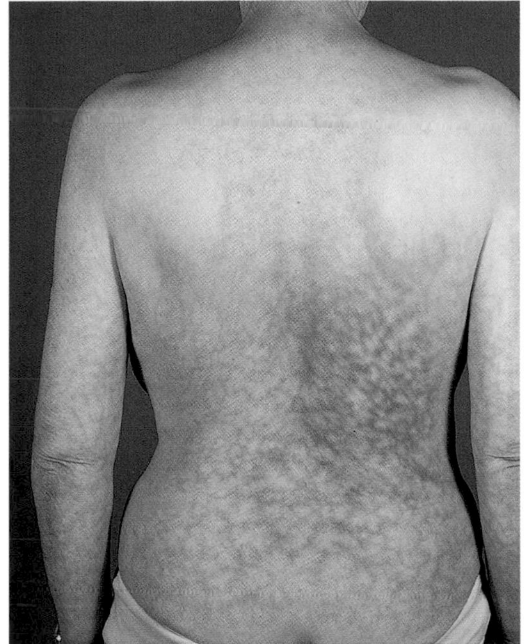

Fig. 82 Erythema ab igne in a patient with chronic pancreatitis.

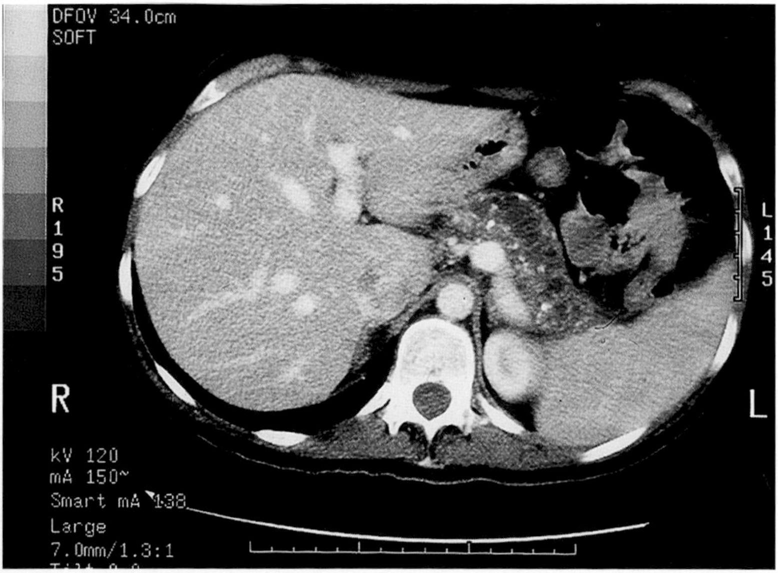

Fig. 83 CT scan showing calcification in the pancreas and a dilated pancreatic duct, which are characteristic features of chronic pancreatitis.

32 Umbilical pathology

Umbilical fistula/sinus

Definition

Failure of the vitello-intestinal duct or urachus to become obliterated are rare causes of discharge from the umbilicus. The vitello-intestinal duct connects the umbilicus to the terminal ileum and, if it remains patent throughout its length, intestinal contents will discharge. The urachus connects the bladder to the umbilicus and if it remains patent a urinary fistula may develop. Either duct may remain patent only at the umbilical end, to form a blind sinus that discharges mucus (Fig. 84).

Clinical features

Persistent discharge is the principal symptom and this may be associated with excoriation of the surrounding skin.

Differential diagnosis

In an infant, umbilical discharge may be caused by an umbilical granuloma following infection of the umbilical cord stump. In adults, umbilical infection with discharge may result from poor hygiene, but an underlying sinus or fistulous tract should be excluded.

Management

Persistent discharge or repeated infections may require excision of the sinus tract or umbilical fistula. Excision of the entire umbilicus may be required.

Malignant nodules of the umbilicus

Secondary carcinoma may present as a hard nodule at the umbilicus (Sister Joseph's nodule; Fig. 85). It is frequently associated with advanced intra-abdominal malignancy, e.g. pancreatic, colon, stomach or ovarian cancer.

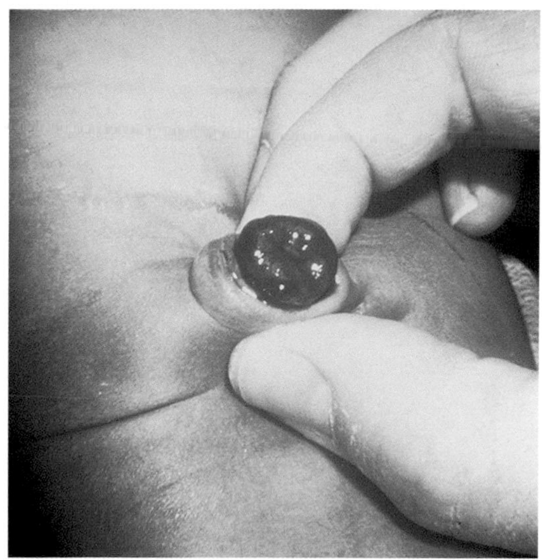

Fig. 84 Umbilical fistula in a child with a Meckel's diverticulum.

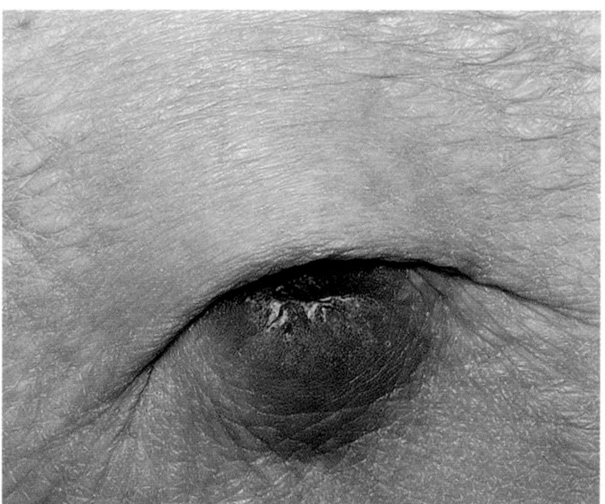

Fig. 85 Sister Joseph's nodule (metastatic carcinoma involving the umbilicus).

33 Ventral hernia

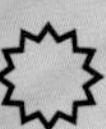

Definition — A hernia is a swelling caused by protrusion of part or all of an organ through an abnormal defect in the surrounding coverings or tissues.

Incidence — Herniations through the linea alba can be found in 1% of the population from adolescence onwards. Males are three times more commonly affected than females and the protrusions are multiple in 20% of patients.

Classification — Ventral hernias occur through areas of weakness in the anterior abdominal wall, such as the linea alba (epigastric hernia), the umbilicus (umbilical and para-umbilical hernia), and the lateral border of the rectus sheath (spigelian hernia). Protrusion of extraperitoneal fat may be followed by the formation of a peritoneal sac and omentum may enter this, although it is rare for bowel to be found in epigastric hernia.

Clinical features — Most epigastric hernias are asymptomatic and are found incidentally on physical examination; however they may cause local discomfort. Examination reveals a palpable midline swelling, which is usually tender and irreducible. Strangulation is rare.

Management — Symptomatic hernias require surgical repair. Herniated fat is excised and, if a sac is present, the contents are reduced and the sac is excised. The fascial defect is repaired with interrupted non-absorbable sutures.

Other hernias

Spigelian hernia occurs through the linea semilunaris at the outer border of the rectus abdominis muscle. The treatment is surgical repair as the hernia is liable to strangulate.

Lumbar hernia presents as a diffuse bulge above the iliac crest, between the posterior borders of the external oblique and latissimus dorsi muscles. It seldom requires treatment.

Obturator hernia is rare. It is more common in woman than men and may present with knee pain owing to pressure on the obturator nerve. The diagnosis is often only made at laparotomy following strangulation.

Divarication of the recti

This is not a true hernia but involves the rectus abdominis muscles being splayed apart, often as a result of pregnancy or obesity, leaving the central anterior abdominal wall devoid of muscular support. It generally causes no symptoms and requires no treatment. It can be demonstrated by asking the supine patient to lift both heels from the bed (Figs 86, 87).

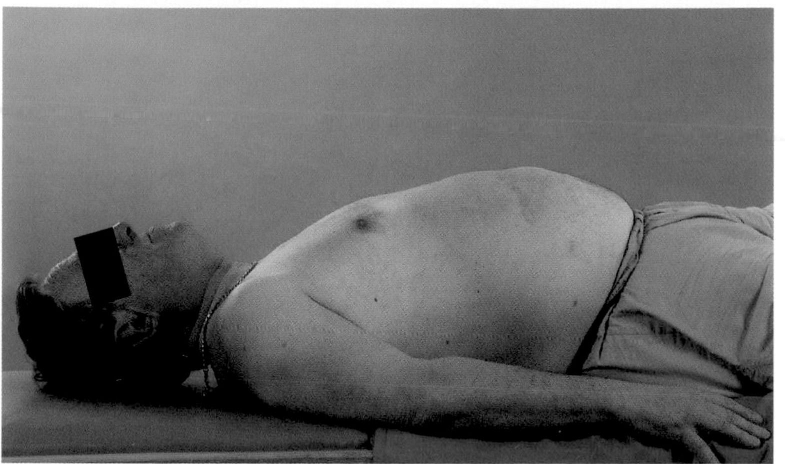

Fig. 86 Bilateral subcostal scar and associated small incisional hernia with marked divarication of the recti. Completely asymptomatic, the abnormalities are not apparent when the patient is supine.

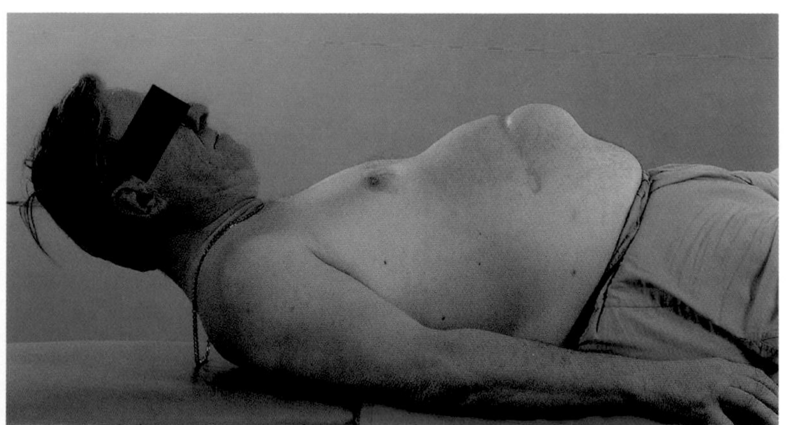

Fig. 87 Lifting his head from the couch reveals marked distortion of the anterior abdominal wall predominately due to the divarication.

34 Umbilical/para-umbilical hernia

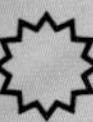

Congenital umbilical hernia

Clinical features

Many new born babies have an umbilical hernia, particularly if premature (Fig. 88). The small sac protrudes through the umbilicus, particularly as the child cries, but is easily reduced. Over 90% of these hernias close spontaneously in the first 3 years of life. Those that remain after that age should be repaired as there is little chance of further improvement.

Management

Surgery is undertaken through a small subumbilical incision. The peritoneal sac is emptied, ligated and excised. The defect in the fascia of the abdominal wall is closed using non-absorbable sutures and the umbilicus is sutured to the repair to restore its normal recessed cosmetic appearance.

Acquired para-umbilical hernia

Definition

This hernia occurs through the linea alba usually just above (or less commonly below) the umbilicus (Fig. 89).

Clinical features

There is local discomfort and a swelling. The emerging sac displaces the umbilical scar, which usually lies below and slightly to one side, resulting in a crescent shape to the umbilicus. The hernia is initially reducible and there may be a palpable defect. It may gradually enlarge with stretching and thinning of the overlying covering tissues. Eventually loops of bowel may become visible under parchment-like skin and the hernia may become irreducible because of adhesions forming between omentum and loops of bowel. Intertrigo may affect the skin and occasionally necrosis may result in development of a fistula.

Differential diagnosis

- Cyst of the vitello-intestinal duct (rare).
- Cyst of the urachus (rare)
- Metastatic tumour deposit (uncommon)

Management

There is a high risk of obstruction and strangulation and therefore repair should be advised even if the hernia is asymptomatic. Most surgical repairs can be performed preserving the umbilicus. Through a transverse subumbilical incision the sac is mobilized, its contents are reduced and the neck of the sac is closed. The abdominal wall is repaired by overlapping its fascial layers using a classical Mayo-type repair. If apposition of the hernia edges is not possible, a non-absorbable mesh can be used.

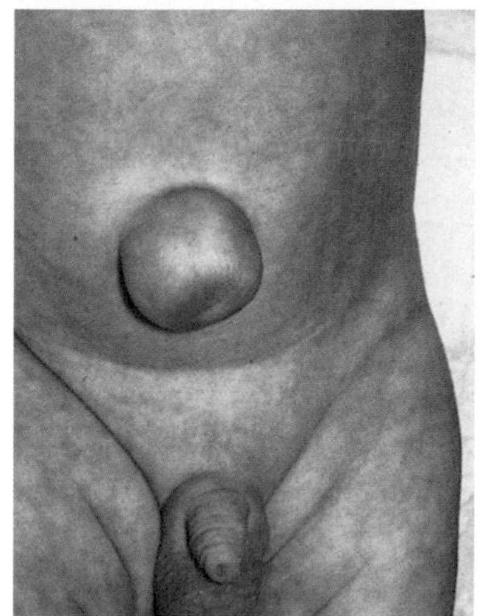

Fig. 88 Umbilical hernia.

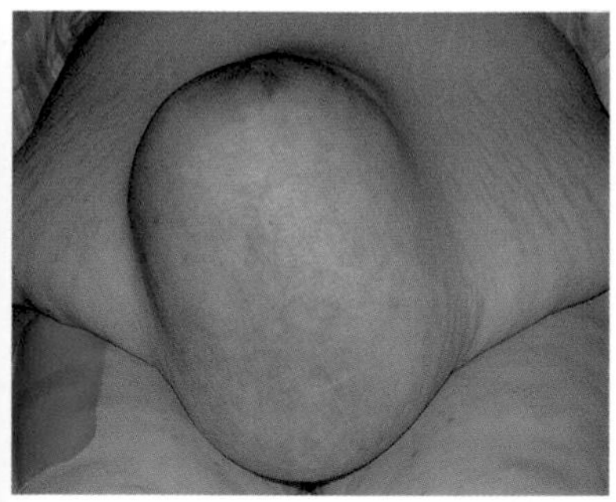

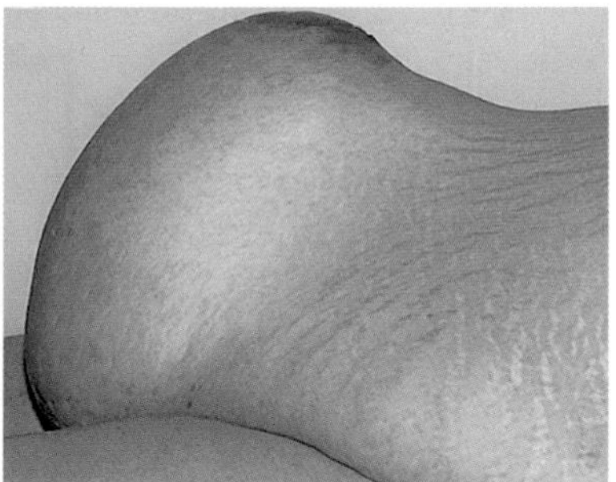

Fig. 89 A&B Large para-umbilical hernia.

35 Incisional hernia

Definition	This can occur in any surgical wound and is a diffuse protrusion of the peritoneum and abdominal contents through a weakened area in the scar.
Incidence	An incisional hernia occurs after 3–5% of all abdominal operations. Midline vertical incisions are most often affected. Poor surgical technique, wound infection, obesity, jaundice, steroid therapy and postoperative chest infection are important predisposing factors. Approximately 40% of incisional hernias occur after a documented wound infection. Most incisional hernias develop within 1 year of an operation and it is unusual for a previously sound closure to become herniated after 3 years. Once a hernia has formed, mechanical forces ensure that it gradually enlarges in size.
Clinical features	The principal symptom is of a bulge in the region of a surgical scar pronounced by coughing (Figs 90, 91). The hernia may cause local discomfort and the overlying skin may become thin and atrophic. Symptoms of intestinal obstruction may develop.
Management	Strangulation is rare; however surgical repair is usually advised even if the incisional hernia is asymptomatic. Protracted observation simply allows the hernia to increase in size, making subsequent repair more difficult and hazardous. The superficial scar is excised and dissection exposes the aponeurosis. The sac can be invaginated and the edges of the defect repaired with an overlapping direct suture technique, but more often a synthetic mesh is inserted (Fig. 92).
Prognosis	The results of surgery for incisional hernia is not as for primary hernias. Small incisional hernias have a recurrence rate of 2–5%, whereas larger hernias have a recurrence rate of 10–20%.

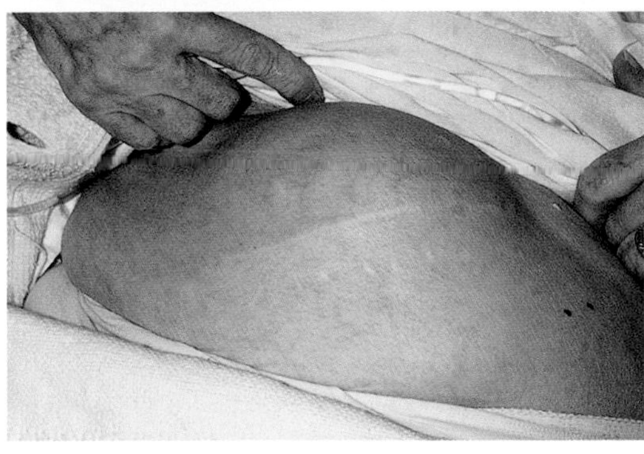

Fig. 90 Incisional hernia.

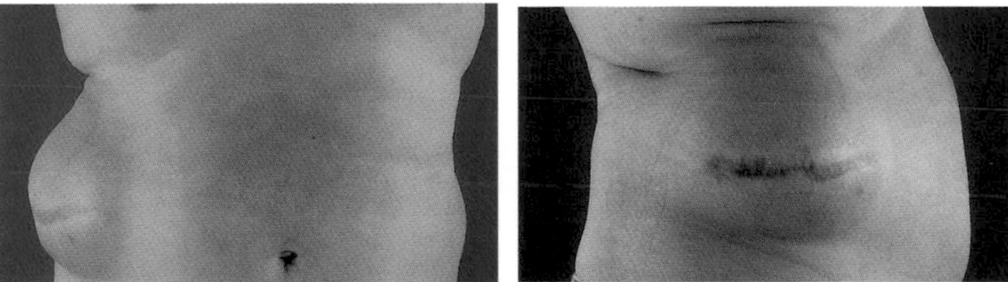

Fig. 91A&B Incisional hernia of a right flank wound following exploration for a sub-hepatic abscess.

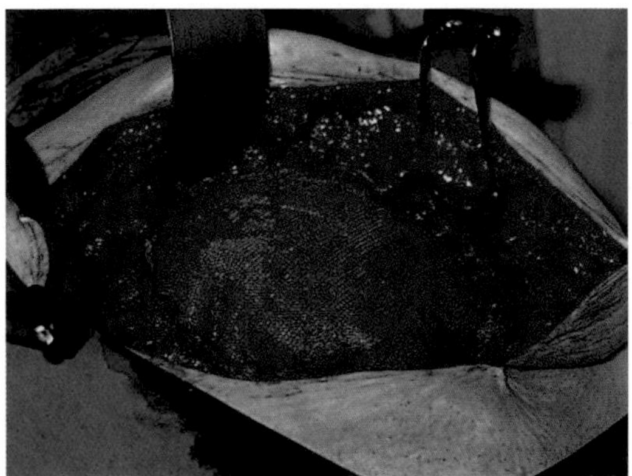

Fig. 92 Large incisional hernia undergoing repair with insertion of a Prolene mesh.

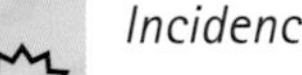

36 Inguinal hernia

Incidence

Groin hernias account for 75–80% of all abdominal hernias. Inguinal hernias are 10 times more common in men than in women. They can occur at any age but are more common before the age of 5 and after middle age. A smaller peak occurs in the early twenties and probably result from a congenital predisposition exacerbated by work or sport.

Classification

- Indirect inguinal hernia
- Direct inguinal hernia
- Pantaloon hernia (combination of both an indirect and direct inguinal hernia)

Clinical features

The moment of herniation (or rupture) may be associated with sudden groin pain, or may pass unnoticed. Thereafter there may be discomfort in the groin. A swelling forms, which may reduce spontaneously when the patient lies flat or after gentle manipulation (Figs 93, 94). An indirect inguinal hernia may be controlled by placing a finger over the deep inguinal ring. It may be necessary to stand the patient up to detect a small hernia. Coughing may result in a visible protrusion of the swelling or be palpated as a cough impulse.

Differential diagnosis

- Femoral hernia
- Lipoma of the spermatic cord
- Encysted hydrocele of the cord
- Undescended or ectopic testis
- Inguinal lymph node
- Saphena varix

Management

All children with an inguinal hernia (Fig. 95) should undergo surgery. In newborns the procedure must be carried out with some urgency because of the risk of incarceration. Most adults with an inguinal hernia require an operation. A truss can be applied in frail elderly patients. Repair can be by an open or laparoscopic technique; the latter is particularly useful in patients with recurrent or bilateral inguinal hernias.

Complications

An enlarging hernia may become irreducible, although this is not an indication for an urgent operation. An inguinal hernia may cause bowel obstruction and, if a hernia strangulates, it becomes tense, tender, irreducible and transmits no impulse on coughing. An obstructed or strangulated hernia requires emergency operation.

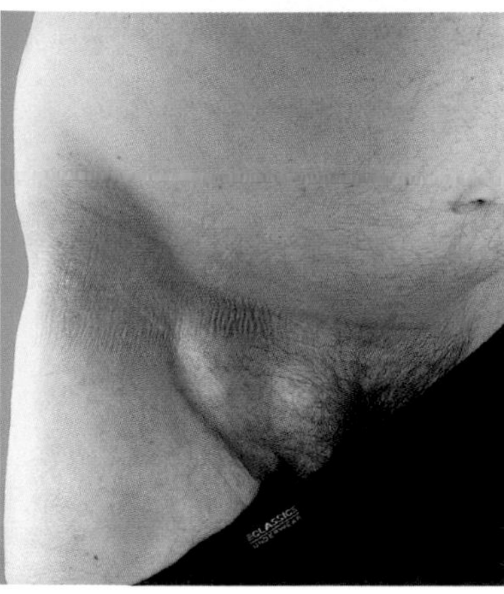

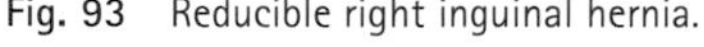

Fig. 93 Reducible right inguinal hernia.

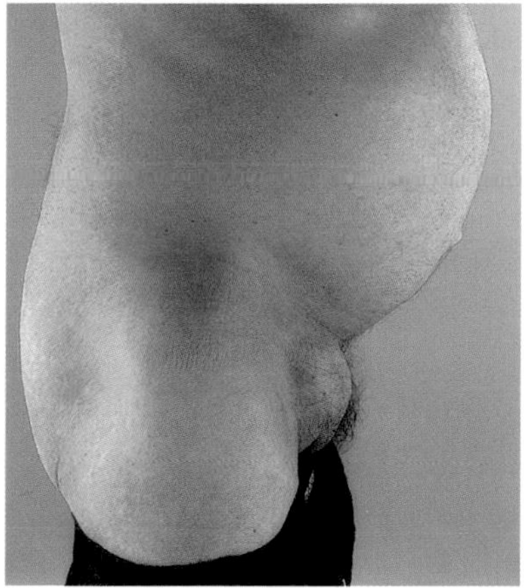

Fig. 94 Lateral view of patient with moderate ascites due to advanced liver cirrhosis and reducible right inguinal hernia.

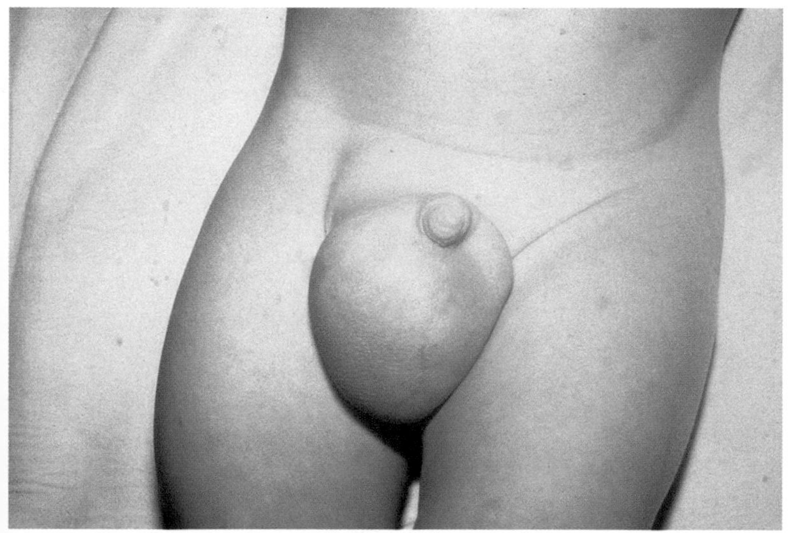

Fig. 95 Paediatric inguinal hernia.

37 Femoral hernia

Definition

Femoral hernias are acquired downward protrusions of peritoneum into the potential space of the femoral canal.

Incidence

Femoral hernias are four times more common in women than men and account for a third of all groin hernias in females (5% in men). They are most common in late middle age and in the multiparous. Unlike inguinal hernias, femoral hernias are rare in children. Bilateral femoral hernias occur in 20%.

Clinical features

The history is often that of an intermittent lump low in the groin; however, frequently the first presentation is with strangulation. A femoral hernia emerges through the femoral ring below and lateral to the pubic tubercle. As the femoral ring is small and unyielding, femoral hernias have a particular tendency to become irreducible, causing strangulation or bowel obstruction (Fig. 96). Sometimes only part of the bowel circumference is strangulated (Richter's hernia) so infarction/strangulation of the wall can occur without signs of obstruction.

Differential diagnosis

- Lipoma in the femoral canal
- An enlarged Cloquet's lymph node

Management

All femoral hernias, even if asymptomatic, should be repaired without delay because of their great risk of strangulation. There is no role for the use of a truss in the management of femoral hernias. Repair is performed by emptying and excising the peritoneal sac. The femoral canal is then closed with non-absorbable sutures. A high approach gives the best access in the emergency situation and is particularly useful if the hernia contains strangulated bowel requiring intestinal resection.

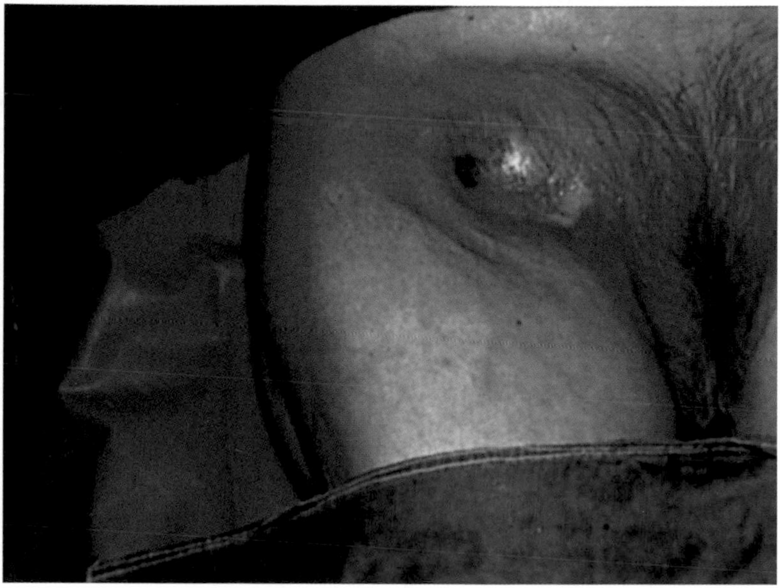

A

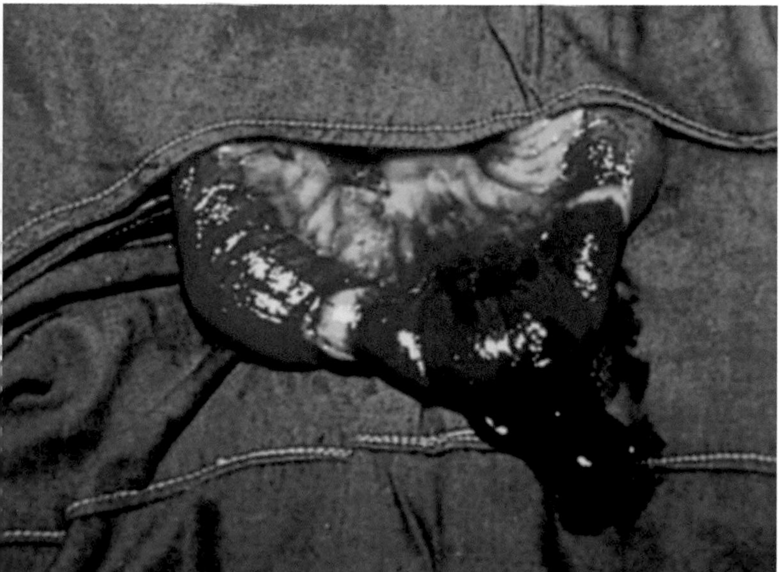

B

Fig. 96 Irreducible femoral hernia containing ischaemic ileum and gangrenous Meckel's diverticulum. The white rings around the bowel (B) are ischaemic in nature and the patient required a small bowel resection and primary anastomosis.

38 Groin lesions

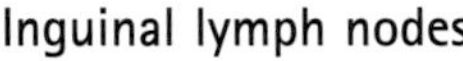

Inguinal lymph nodes

Inguinal lymph nodes drain the lower abdominal wall, lower back, perineum, anal canal, penis and lower limbs and may become secondarily enlarged as a result of conditions affecting this region. Examples include infections of the foot, skin diseases, sexually transmitted infection or tumours. Inguinal lymph node enlargement may be part of a generalized lymphadenopathy due to lymphoma or systemic infection. Enlarged inguinal lymph nodes may present with pain, but often they are an incidental finding. Fine-needle aspiration cytology or excisional biopsy may establish the diagnosis.

Saphena varix

A saphena varix is a dilatation of the long saphenous vein in the groin just distal to an incompetent saphenofemoral valve (Fig. 97). It is caused by the high pressure of venous blood in the upright posture and is usually associated with varicose veins elsewhere in the long saphenous system. The varix can present as a prominent bulge and can reach the size of a golf ball or even larger. The bulge disappears when the patient lies down and can be easily emptied with minimal pressure in the upright position. A cough impulse is invariably present and a thrill may be palpated by tapping on the long saphenous vein in the thigh. Treatment is high saphenous ligation (Fig. 98).

Femoral artery aneurysm

Femoral artery aneurysm is an uncommon cause of a lump in the groin. It may occur in isolation but is more often part of a generalized aneurysmal disease affecting other major blood vessels. The lump lies below the mid point of the inguinal ligament and has a characteristic expansile pulsation.

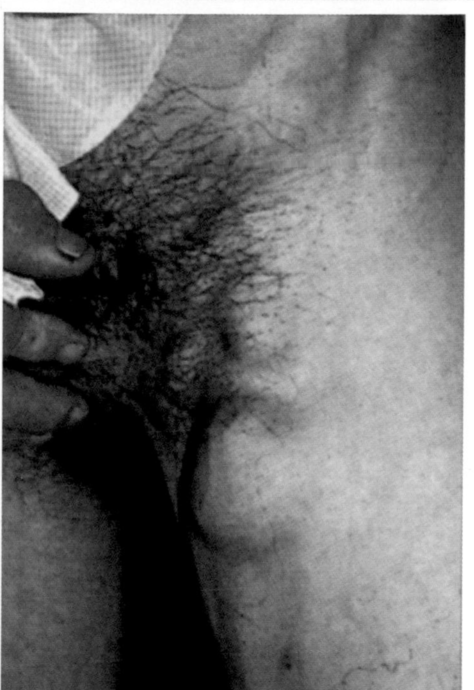

Fig. 97 Saphena varix. This is a 'blow out' at the saphenofemoral junction.

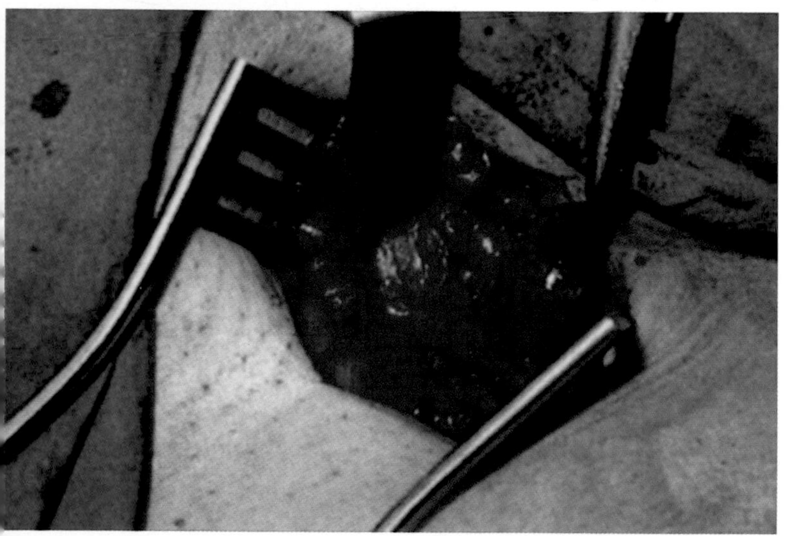

Fig. 98 Standard treatment of saphena varix is ligation at the saphenofemoral junction with above knee stripping of the long saphenous vein.

39 Hydrocele

Definition

An excessive collection of fluid within the tunica vaginalis (the serous space surrounding the testis).

Classification

- Congenital – most will resolve by the age of 1 year
- Acquired – usually idiopathic, but 10% are associated with tumour or infection of the testis

Clinical features

Hydroceles present as painless scrotal swellings (Fig. 99). The swelling is smooth and transilluminates. The normal testis cannot be palpated and one can get above the swelling, which differentiates it from an inguinal hernia.

Differential diagnosis

- Epididymo-orchitis
- Epididymal cyst
- Varicocele
- Testicular tumour.

Management

Aspiration of fluid alone does not cure an idiopathic hydrocele and the fluid will recollect. It is possible to obliterate the sac by injecting a sclerosant following aspiration, but surgical excision and eversion is associated with a much lower recurrence rate. If the hydrocele fluid becomes infected, incision and drainage of the pus is necessary.

Epididymal cyst

Most cysts develop as a painless scrotal swelling. Epididymal cysts tend to affect a younger age group than hydroceles. The differentiating clinical feature is that an epididymal cyst can be palpated separately from the testis. It tends to lie near the upper pole of the testis and can be transilluminated.

Varicocele

The veins of the pampiniform plexus become dilated and tortuous, producing a swelling in the scrotum that resembles 'a bag of worms'. It is more common on the left side and may be associated with infertility. A dragging sensation in the scrotum may cause concern to the patient. Treatment is by ligation of the spermatic vein, which may be done surgically (laparoscopically) at the internal inguinal ring or radiologically by embolization.

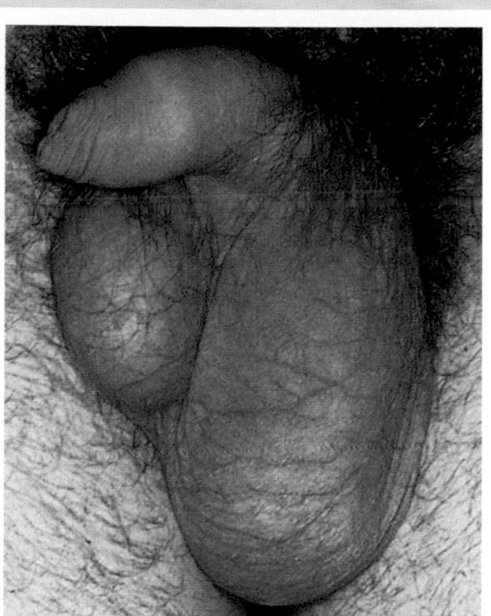

Fig. 99 Hydrocele.

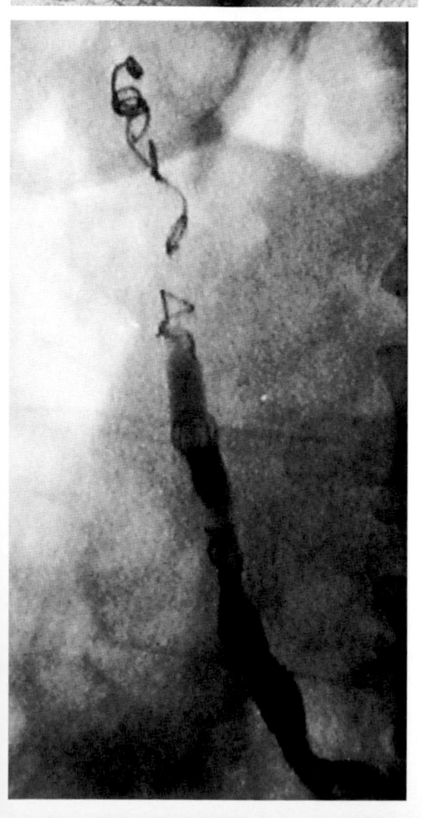

Fig. 100 Embolisation of multiple veins in left varicocele.

40 Testicular tumours

Incidence

Testicular tumours are uncommon, with an incidence of 5/100,000. In males, they comprise about 1% of all malignancies. They most commonly affect men aged between 20 and 40 years of age.

Classification

90% of primary testicular tumours are derived from germ cells; the rest include gonadal, stromal, mesenchymal and ductal tumours. Teratomas (Fig. 101) account for approximately 60% of germ cell tumours and seminomas (Figs 102, 103) approximately 35%.

Clinical features

The commonest presentation is of a progressively enlarging testicular lump. Both seminoma and teratoma spread via lymphatics to para-aortic lymph nodes and then via the lymphatic chain and thoracic duct to the supraclavicular nodes and the systemic circulation. Lung secondaries are particularly common in teratomas. Examination may reveal a hard lump in the body of the testis or diffuse testicular enlargement.

Management

Orchidectomy is performed through a groin incision. In order to reduce the risk of disseminating malignant cells, the spermatic cord is mobilized and clamped before the testis is delivered from the scrotum. Radiotherapy is the treatment of choice for early-stage seminoma, as this tumour is very radio-sensitive. The management of teratoma depends on the stage of the disease, and may include chemotherapy.

Prognosis

The 5-year survival rate for patients with seminoma is 90–95%. The more variable prognosis of teratomas depends on tumour type, stage and volume. For more favourable tumours the 5-year survival rate may be as high as 95%, but in more advanced cases 5-year survival of 60–70% is more usual.

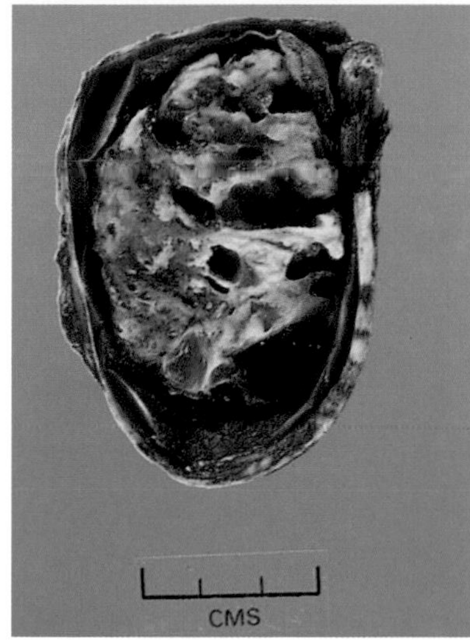

Fig. 101 Teratoma. This lesion arises from primitive germinal cells and thus may contain cartilage, bone, muscle, fat and other tissues.

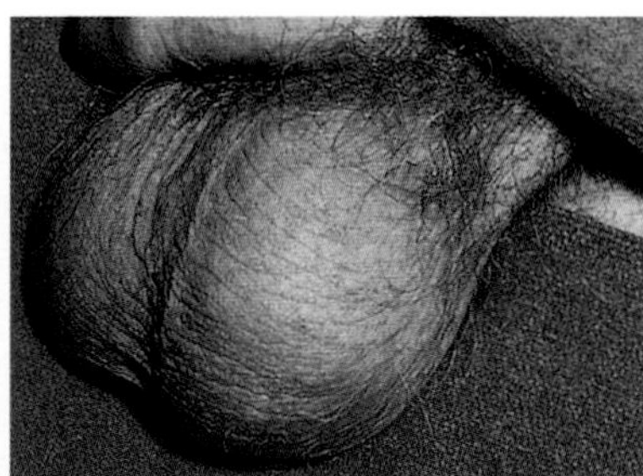

Fig. 102 Seminoma in a 35-year old man.

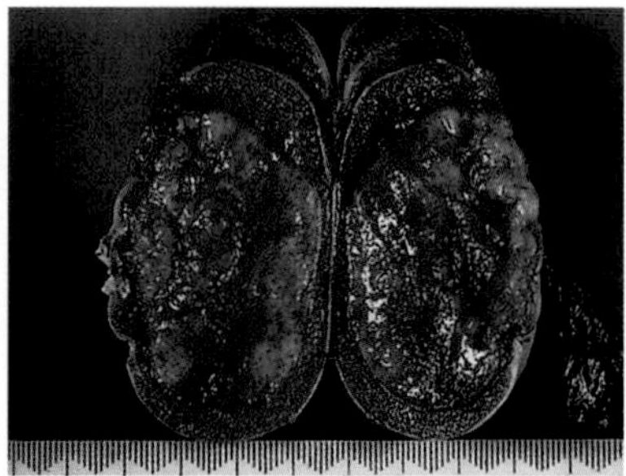

Fig. 103 The cut surface of a seminoma demonstrating a rather amorphous, pale appearance.

41 Testicular torsion

Aetiology

Torsion is a recognized complication of testicular maldescent and is rare after adolescence.

Clinical features

There may be a history of previous self-limiting episodes of testicular pain. Testicular torsion presents with a sudden onset of severe testicular pain often accompanied by vague central abdominal pain and vomiting. In the early stages of torsion, the affected testis is tender, slightly swollen and drawn up into the neck of the scrotum, where the cord may be palpably thickened (Fig. 104). On examination there is a red, swollen hemiscrotum that is usually too tender to palpate.

Differential diagnosis

- Torsion of an epididymal appendage (see below)
- Acute epididymo-orchitis
- Idiopathic scrotal oedema.

Management

Torsion of the testis is a surgical emergency requiring prompt diagnosis and urgent surgical treatment if the testis is to be saved. If the blood supply is not restored within 6 hours, infarction ensues and the testis must be excised (Fig. 105).

Torsion of the epididymal appendage (hydatid of Morgagni)

A small embryological remnant on the upper pole of the testis is known as the hydatid of Morgagni. This may undergo torsion and produce symptoms similar to those of testicular torsion. It is often only apparent at surgical exploration when the lesion can be excised.

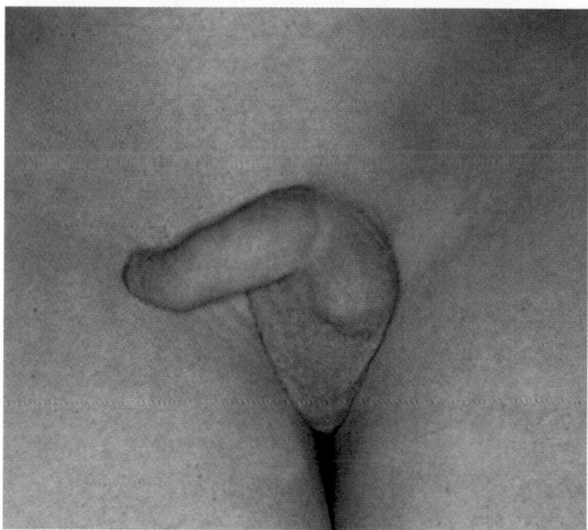

Fig. 104 Testicular torsion. The patient presents with an acutely tender, swollen testis lying high within the scrotum with an abnormal orientation.

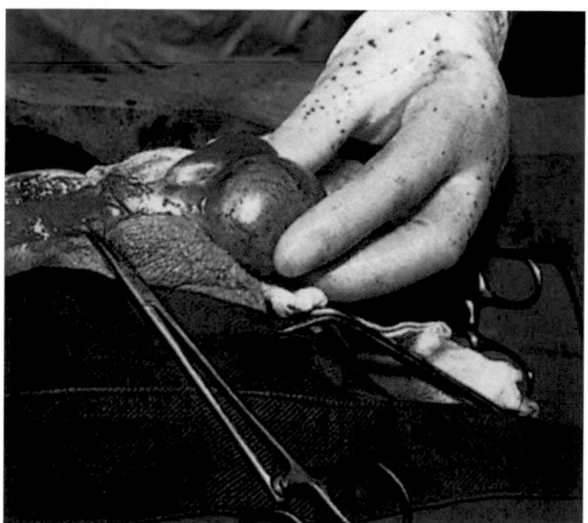

Fig. 105 Emergency exploration of the scrotum is mandatory. At operation a 360% torsion was found, with associated testicular infarction.

42 Disorders of the foreskin

Balanitis

Definition

Balanitis is an inflammation of the glans penis and foreskin commonly caused by *Candida* or faecal bacteria. Balanitis xerotica obliterans is a fibrotic condition of the foreskin of unknown aetiology. It produces a thickened, stenotic, often depigmented foreskin that is frequently adherent to the glans.

Management

Circumcision solves the problem but the process can involve the urethral meatus, causing meatal stenosis and sometimes may require meatotomy or meatoplasty at the same time.

Phimosis

Definition

This is an inability to retract the foreskin (Fig. 106).

Classification

Phimosis may be congenital or acquired. The latter may develop as a result of recurrent balanitis or because of an underlying tumour of the glans penis.

Clinical features

The preputial orifice is white, scarred and indurated. Presenting symptoms include inability to retract the foreskin, irritation or bleeding exacerbated by sexual intercourse.

Management

Treatment is by circumcision. The operation should not be undertaken if infection is present.

Paraphimosis

Definition

If a phimotic foreskin is forcibly retracted, the tight meatal band may lodge in the coronal sulcus, making reduction impossible. Progressive oedema of the glans penis and foreskin then exacerbates the difficulty of reduction (Fig. 107).

Management

Local anaesthetic jelly is applied first for lubrication and pain relief. Gentle pressure and traction will often reduce the foreskin. Sometimes it may be necessary to incise the tight foreskin under local or general anaesthesia to effect reduction.

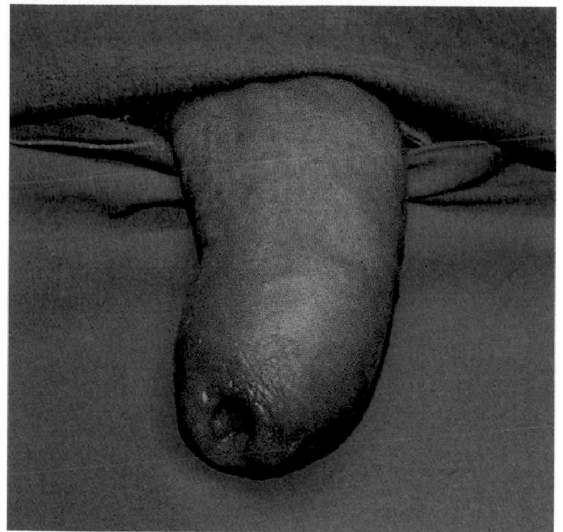

Fig. 106 Phimosis.

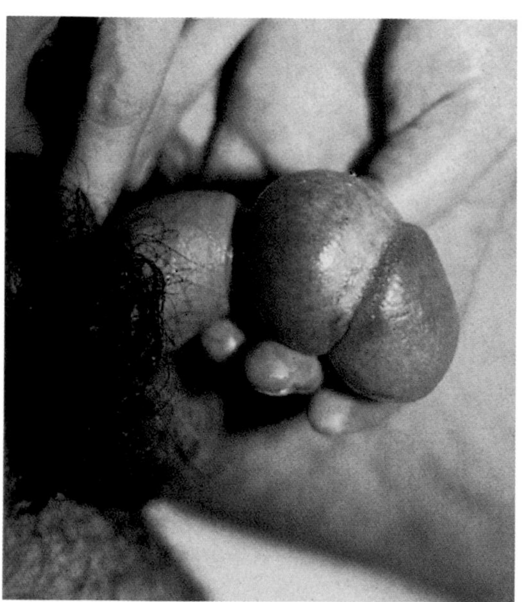

Fig. 107 Paraphimosis. Poorly retracted foreskin acts as a tight band and causes engorgement of the glans.

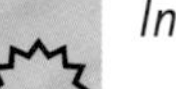

43 Carcinoma of the penis

Incidence

This uncommon tumour has an incidence of 1.5/100 000 and is generally attributed to poor hygiene associated with a non-retractable foreskin. It is very rare in circumcised men and almost always occurs in the elderly. Histologically, the tumours are squamous-cell carcinomas, usually well differentiated, that arise from the inner surface of the foreskin over the glans penis in the region of the coronal sulcus.

Clinical features

The patient may present with a purulent or blood stained discharge issuing from beneath a non-retractile foreskin. The tumour invades locally and unfortunately many patients do not seek help until the lesion is advanced (Figs 108, 109). On occasions much of the penis is already destroyed and the inguinal lymph nodes are involved.

Management

Circumcision may cure early tumours confined to the prepuce. Small tumours confined to the glans may be treated by excision of the glans and skin grafting. Advanced tumours require partial or total penile amputation and often bilateral block dissection of inguinal lymph nodes. Inoperable tumours are treated by radiotherapy.

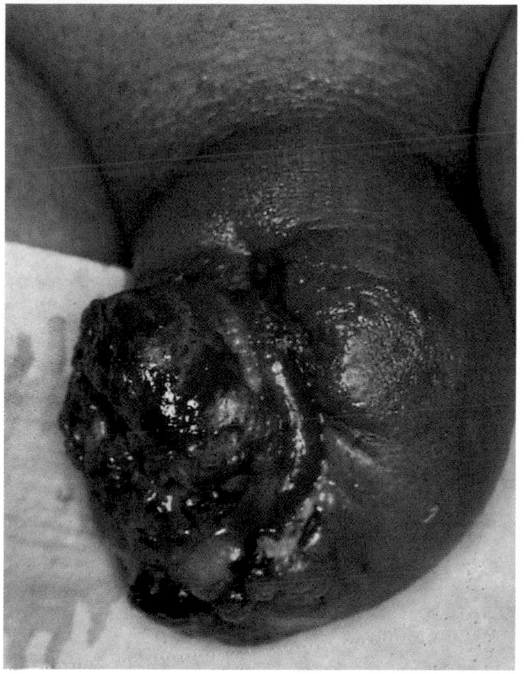

Fig. 108 Carcinoma of the penis.

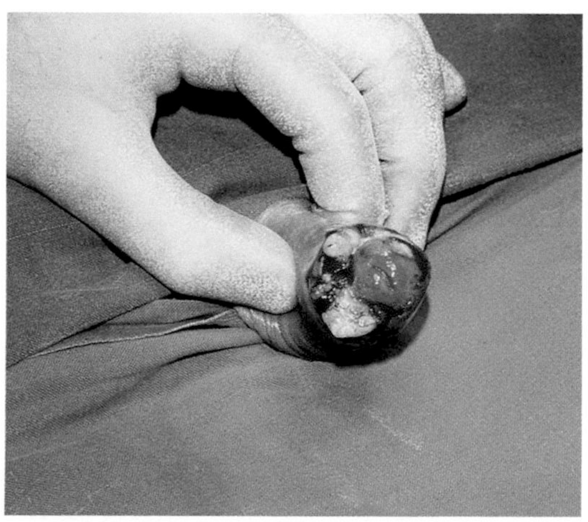

Fig. 109 Carcinoma of the penis.

44 Hypospadias/epispadias

Hypospadias

Incidence

Hypospadias is a common congenital abnormality of the penis and urethra occurring in approximately 1/400 male births. Failure of the embryonic folds to fuse results in abnormal placing of the external urinary meatus on the ventral surface of the penis (Fig. 110).

Clinical features

The urethral meatus may lie anywhere along the penile shaft or in the perineum. The remnant of urethra tissue distal to the meatus is fibrotic, causing the penis to bend downwards on erection, this is known as chordee. In addition, the ventral part of the foreskin is absent, giving rise to a hooded appearance.

Management

Repair is a highly specialized procedure and utilizes the hood of the foreskin. The aim is to construct a new urethral opening in the normal position on the glans. Circumcision should never be carried out without specialist advice.

Epispadias

In this condition the external urinary meatus opens on the dorsal surface of the penis. It is much less common than hypospadias and may be associated with other major genito-urinary abnormalities. The mucosa of the bladder and ureteric orifices may be exposed and form the infra-umbilical part of the abdominal wall (exstrophy; Fig. 111). Reconstruction of these deformities is not always successful and urinary incontinence may remain a major problem and require urinary diversion.

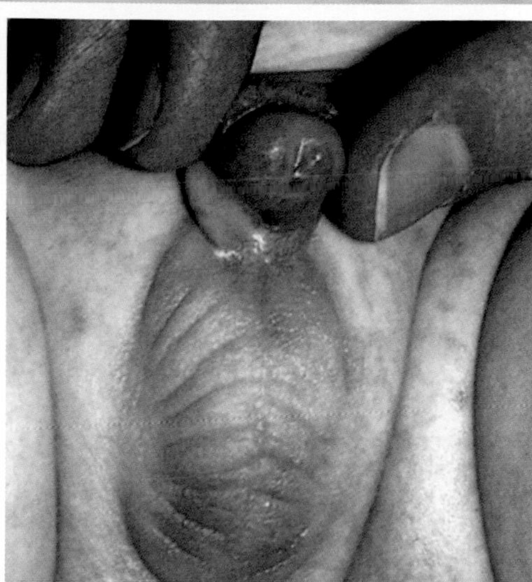

Fig. 110 Glandular hypospadias.

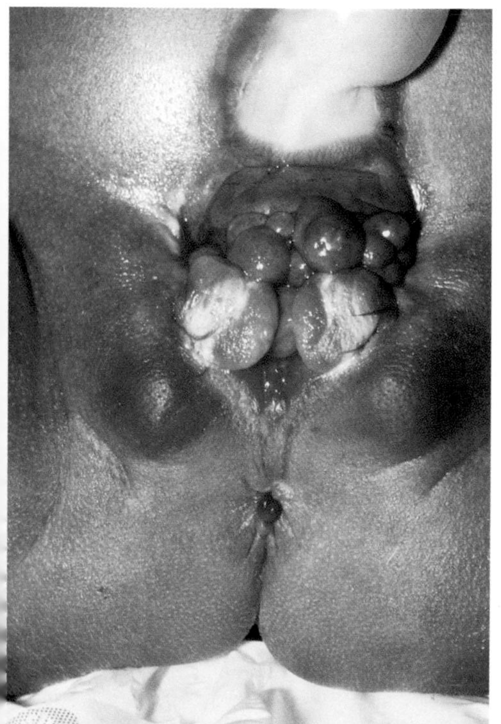

Fig. 111 Ectopia vesicae is an uncommon congenital malformation where the bladder mucosa is exposed to the anterior abdominal wall.

45 Haemorrhoids

Definition

Haemorrhoids are enlarged prolapsed anal cushions resulting from degeneration and stretching of the supporting fibroelastic tissue and smooth muscle.

Incidence

Haemorrhoids are extremely common, affecting nearly half of the population at some stage in their lives. Men tend to suffer more often, whereas women are particularly susceptible in late pregnancy and during the puerperium.

Classification

- First-degree haemorrhoids – never prolapse
- Second-degree haemorrhoids – prolapse during defaecation but reduce spontaneously
- Third-degree haemorrhoids – remain outside the anal margin unless replaced digitally.

Most haemorrhoids can be described as 'internal' because they are covered by glandular mucosa. Large neglected haemorrhoids may extend beneath the stratified squamous epithelium so that their lower part becomes covered by skin ('external' haemorrhoids).

Clinical features

Bleeding and prolapse are the cardinal features. The bleeding is typically intermittent, fresh blood that is separate from stool and evident in the pan or only on wiping. There may also be aching or dragging on defaecation. Perianal irritation and itching (pruritus ani) may be a feature. The appearance may vary from slightly enlarged anal cushions visible only at proctoscopy to large external haemorrhoids (Figs 112, 113). Thrombosed or strangulated haemorrhoids present with acute pain and may require hospital admission. They are usually obvious on inspection as oedematous, congested purplish masses. Tight spasm of the anal sphincter makes digital rectal examination extremely painful.

Management

- Laxatives to prevent constipation
- Rubber band ligation
- Injection sclerotherapy
- Infra-red photocoagulation
- Haemorrhoidectomy

Perianal haematoma

This is a painful condition caused by thrombus in the subcutaneous superficial space in the perianal region. The clinical appearance is of a discrete, blue-coloured swelling that has the appearance of a small blackcurrant. It may resolve with symptomatic management; however deroofing the lesion gives instantaneous relief.

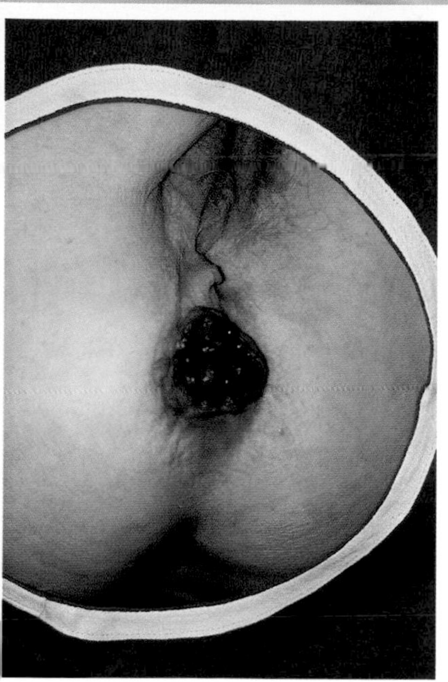

Fig. 112 Prolapsing haemorrhoids.

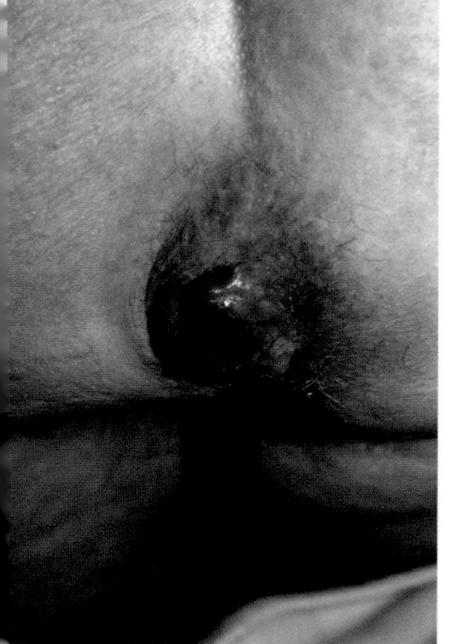

Fig. 113 Prolapsing haemorrhoids with descending perineum.

46 Anal fissure

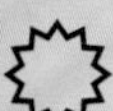

Definition

An anal fissure is a longitudinal tear in the mucosa and skin of the anal canal (Figs 114, 115). The commonest site is posteriorly in the midline but it may be anterior or lateral. The condition most commonly affects people in their 20s and 30s, with a slight male preponderance.

Aetiology

They are usually caused by passing a large constipated stool but may be secondary to anal intercourse.

Clinical features

Pain is the predominant feature. It is exacerbated by defaecation and may be severe. The pain may continue for several hours before easing until the next stool, when the cycle is repeated. Constipation may ensue as a consequence of the patient's unwillingness to defaecate because of pain. Bleeding is not usually severe and may occur only on the toilet paper after defaecation. An anal fissure is described as chronic when it has an ulcer at the base and has been present for at least 6 weeks. The fissure may be concealed by anal spasm, but a small skin tag (sentinel pile) may be seen superficially. Rectal examination is extremely painful and rarely possible.

Differential diagnosis

- Crohn's disease
- Primary syphilitic chancre
- Herpes simplex
- Neoplasia
- Ruptured perianal haematoma.

Management

Conservative management involves the use of topical glyceryl trinitrate (GTN) ointment 0.2% applied topically. This treatment can cure up to 60% of anal fissures but may be associated with headaches. Surgery in the form of a lateral submucous (internal) sphincterotomy usually gives immediate relief but there is a 10–15% incidence of incontinence of flatus following this procedure. The operation involves controlled division of the lower half of the internal sphincter. The anal stretch procedure has now been abandoned as this was associated with significant sphincter damage and incontinence. Dietary advice regarding fibre intake should be given to help prevent recurrences.

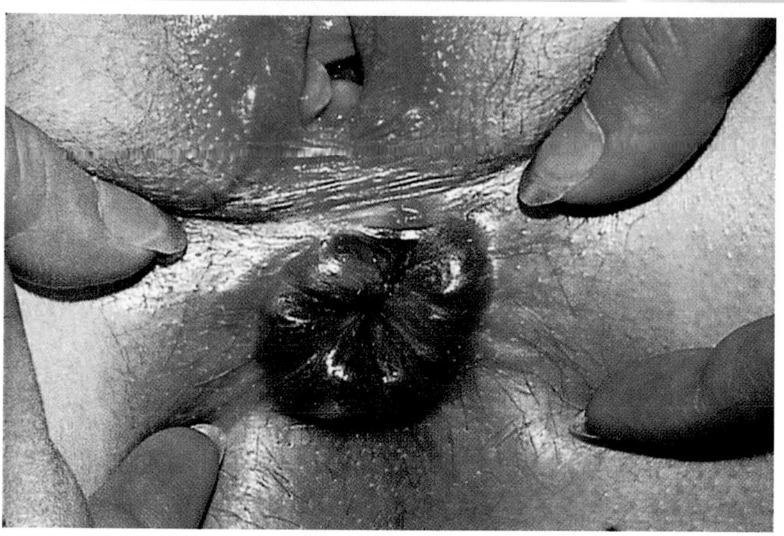

Fig. 114 Anterior anal fissure.

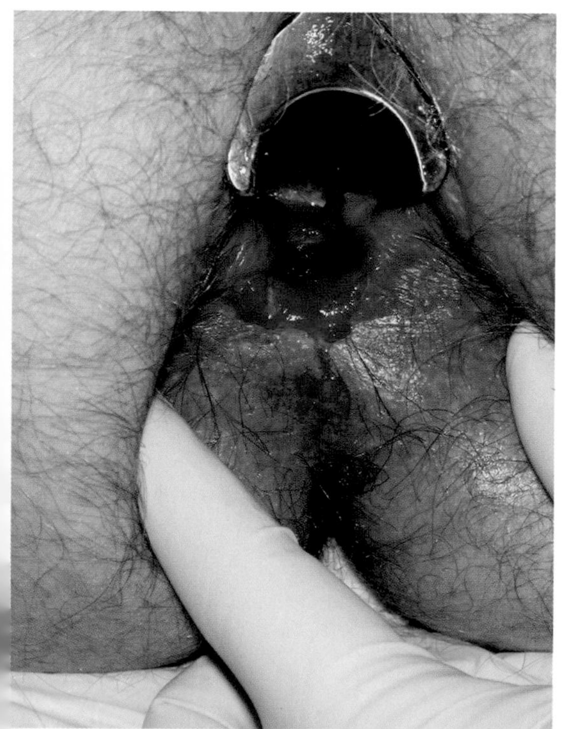

Fig. 115 Large chronic posterior anal fissure.

47 Anorectal abscesses

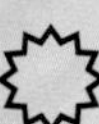

Definition

Anorectal suppuration is common, affecting men three times more frequently than women, and is a common surgical emergency. The abscess is thought to arise in the anal glands, which lie in the intersphincteric plane. If the pus tracks inferiorly, a perianal abscess presents externally (Fig. 116). The pus may also track superiorly to form a pelvirectal abscess or laterally to form an ischiorectal abscess (Fig. 117).

Classification

- Pelvirectal abscess
- High intermuscular abscess
- Intersphincteric abscess
- Ischiorectal abscess – make up about 15% of ano-rectal abscesses.
- Perianal abscess – this is the most common presentation and accounts for 80% of ano-rectal abscesses.

Clinical features

The patient with a perianal abscess presents with a painful tender red swelling close to the anal verge that is clinically obvious on external examination. The deeper abscesses may expand without causing much pain but can produce symptoms of systemic sepsis and deep perineal pain.

Management

Anorectal abscesses require surgical drainage (Fig. 118). Antibiotics are only indicated if there is spreading infection. Perianal and ischiorectal abscesses are drained via the perianal skin, ensuring all loculations are broken down. Large abscess cavities require packing or placement of a drain to keep the neck of the cavity open and the defect is allowed to heal by secondary intention. A significant number of patients develop an anal fistula. Unusually complex perianal sepsis or recurrent abscesses should raise the suspicion of underlying inflammatory bowel disease, particularly Crohn's disease.

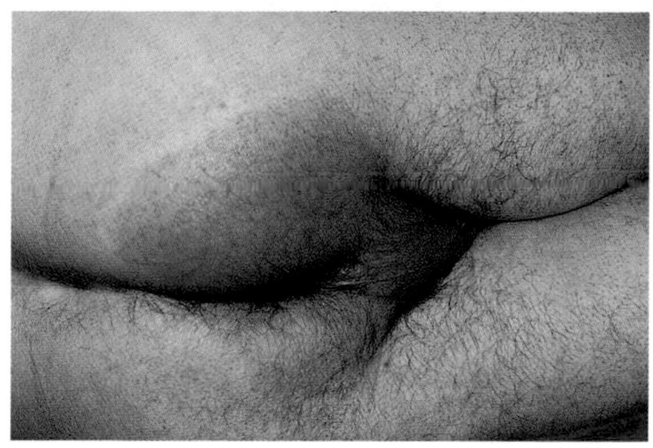

Fig. 116 Perineal abscess.

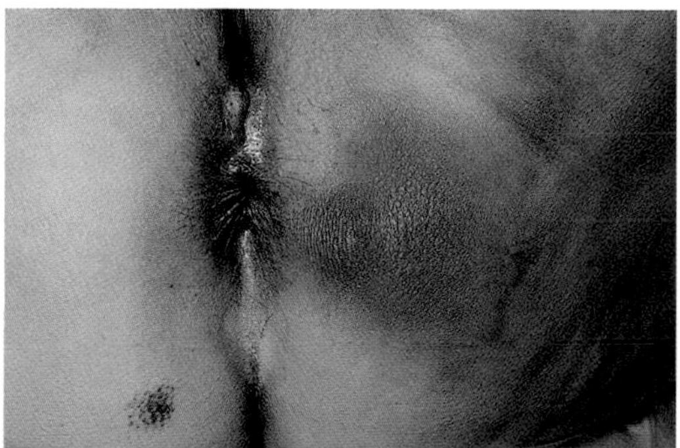

Fig. 117 Ischiorectal abscess.

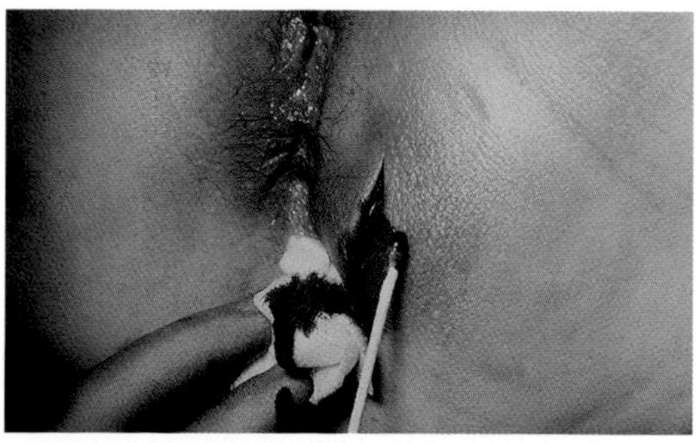

Fig. 118 Incision and drainage of ischiorectal abscess.

48 Anal fistula

Definition

A fistula is an abnormal communication between two epithelial-lined surfaces. An anal fistula is a communication consisting of a chronically infected tract extending from an internal opening, usually at the dentate line, to the perianal skin.

Aetiology

Anal fistulas usually develop as a complication of anorectal sepsis.

Classification

- Intersphincteric – the inflammatory tracts remain medial to the striated muscle
- Trans-sphincteric – the tract breaches the external sphincter
- Supra-sphincteric (rare) – the primary tract passes across the levator ani

Clinical features

The typical complaint is of an intermittent discharge of purulent fluid in the perianal region. There may be associated pruritus ani and staining of underwear. On examination a discharging orifice may be obvious within 2–3 cm of the anal margin. Digital palpation may reveal induration between the orifice and the anal canal in keeping with a subcutaneous tract.

'Goodsall's rule' states that fistulas anterior to an imaginary transverse line across the anus usually have a short direct tract to the anal canal. Those behind this imaginary line will commonly have the opening in the midline and pursue a more torturous course.

Differential diagnosis

Other causes of fistula in the perianal region include Crohn's disease (Fig. 119), radiation, trauma and neoplasia.

Management

Assessment and treatment requires examination under anaesthesia (EUA). A probe is inserted to ascertain the course of the tract, which determines subsequent management (Fig. 120). Options include:

- Laying open a low fistulous tract
- 'Seton' suture/sloop – drains sepsis and if tightened will gradually cut through the sphincters, allowing them to heal
- High anal fistula may require complex surgical intervention.

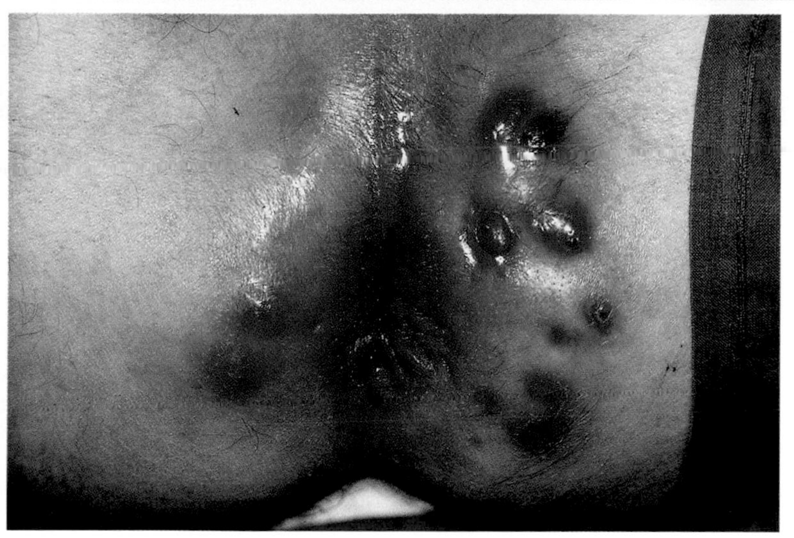

Fig. 119 Multiple anal fistula in association with Crohn's disease.

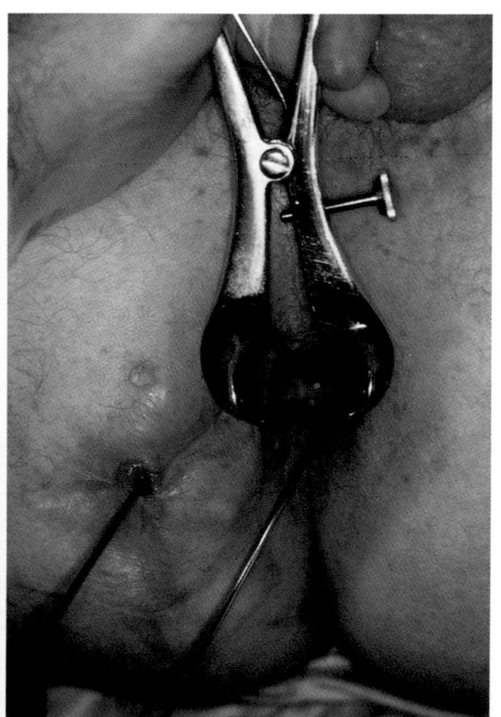

Fig. 120 Recurrent trans-sphincteric anal fistula with probe demonstrating fistulous tract.

49 Pilonidal disease

Definition

A chronic inflammatory condition characterized by the presence of one or more sinuses that contain hair and debris.

Incidence

Pilonidal disease is more common in males than females and affects around 2% of the population between the ages of 15 and 35.

Aetiology

The commonest site for pilonidal disease is the natal cleft (Fig. 121). Other rarer sites include the umbilicus and the webs of the fingers in hairdressers (Fig. 122). Hairs slowly work their way into the dermis, with the cuticular scales on the hairs acting like the barbs of an arrow. The process is encouraged by sitting and sweating. The condition affected large numbers of American servicemen during the Vietnam War owing to the use of jeeps in the warm climate.

Presenting features

Recurrent episodes of pain, tenderness and purulent discharge are the usual presenting features. The characteristic midline pits may have protruding tufts of hair. The surrounding skin may be inflamed or indurated and there may be tenderness on palpation. An abscess may develop, which typically points just off the midline; however, there is invariably a communication with the midline sinus.

Management

No specific treatment is required in asymptomatic patients. Conservative management comprises good hygiene and removal of hair.

There are a number of surgical options for pilonidal sinuses. The tracts can be laid open and curetted followed by dressings allowing the wound to heal by secondary intention. Simple tracts may be excised and closed primarily with sutures, although the wound is prone to breakdown. Surgical drainage is required for an abscess.

Prognosis

Recurrence is common but can be minimized by keeping the natal cleft free of hair. Complex rotational flap procedures can be undertaken.

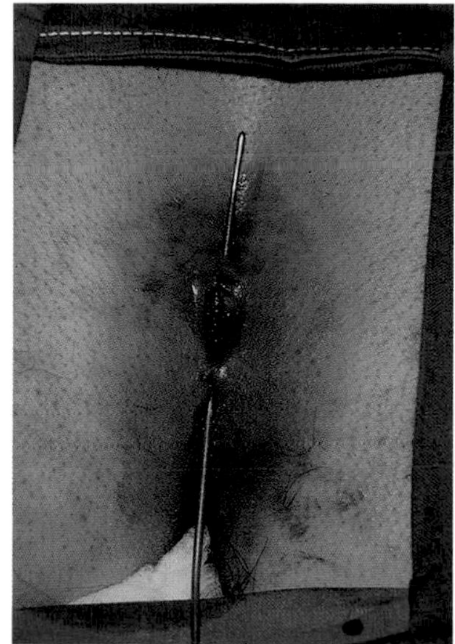

Fig. 121 Pilonidal sinus affecting the natal cleft.

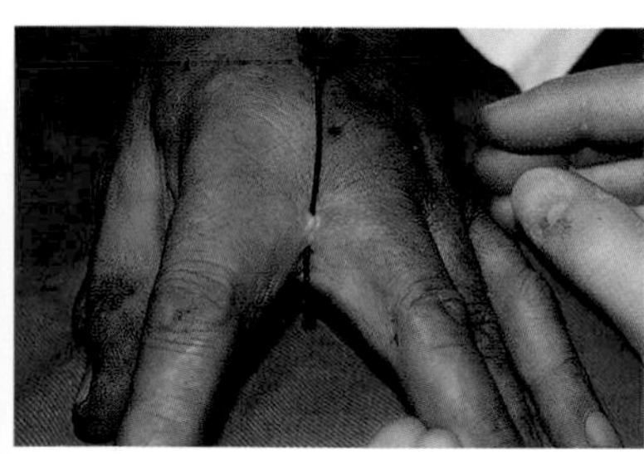

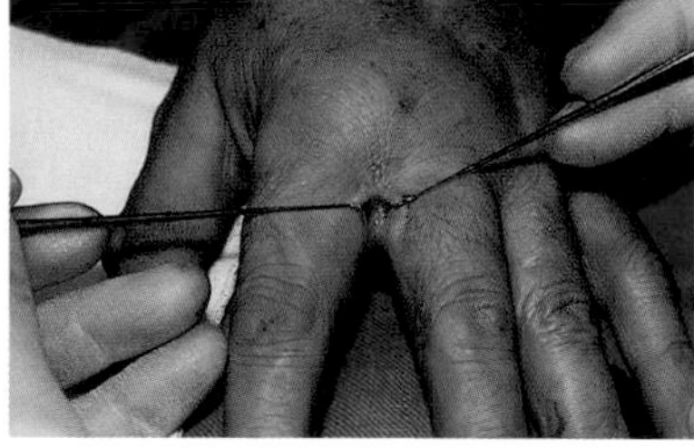

A B

Fig. 122 A&B Pilonidal sinus in the web space between the index and middle finger in a hairdresser.

50 Rectal prolapse

Rectal prolapse is mainly seen in young children and the elderly. In children it is usually a relatively minor and self-correcting problem whereas in the elderly it is a chronic problem.

Classification

- Rectal mucosal prolapse – involves only the mucosa
- Full-thickness rectal prolapse – includes the mucosa and the muscular layers

Clinical features

Patients present with an uncomfortable sensation of 'something coming down' the back passage. Initially, the mass is small and only occurs on defaecation. The size of the prolapse increases with time and eventually the rectal mass remains constantly prolapsed and will not reduce spontaneously (Fig. 123); however the patient may be able to reduce the prolapse digitally. Constipation may initially be an accompanying feature; however, incontinence often develops because of dilatation of the internal anal sphincter. Rectal prolapse is either remarkably well tolerated or else concealed. Hygiene problems may be extremely distressing as the prolapsed bowel secretes mucus, which can irritate the perianal skin. The easily damaged mucosa may bleed on contact. The prolapse may become ulcerated (Fig. 124) and in rare circumstances the rectum may become strangulated. The prolapse may not initially be apparent on examination but straining will usually deliver the prolapse through the anus.

Differential diagnosis

- Third-degree haemorrhoids
- Prolapsing rectal neoplasia
- Anal warts
- Anal skin tags
- Fibroepithelial anal polyp

Management

Surgery is rarely indicated in children. In adults, the surgical approach can be via the abdomen (suture fixation rectopexy or resection rectopexy) or via the perineum (Delorme's procedure or perineal rectosigmoidectomy).

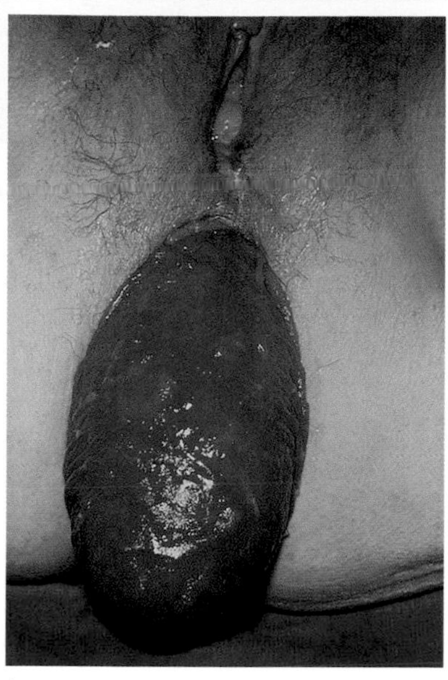

A

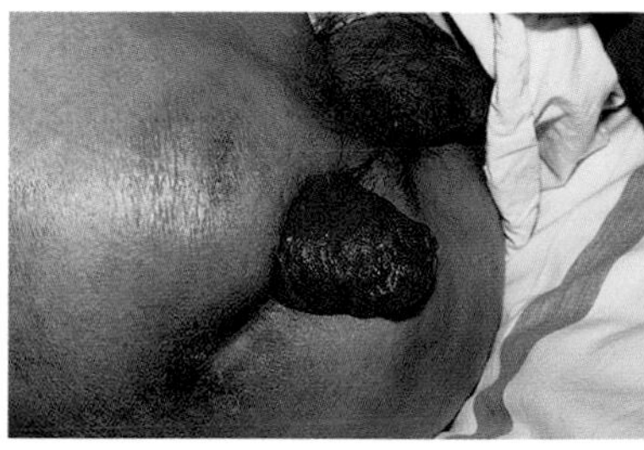

B

Fig. 123 A&B Prolapse of rectum.

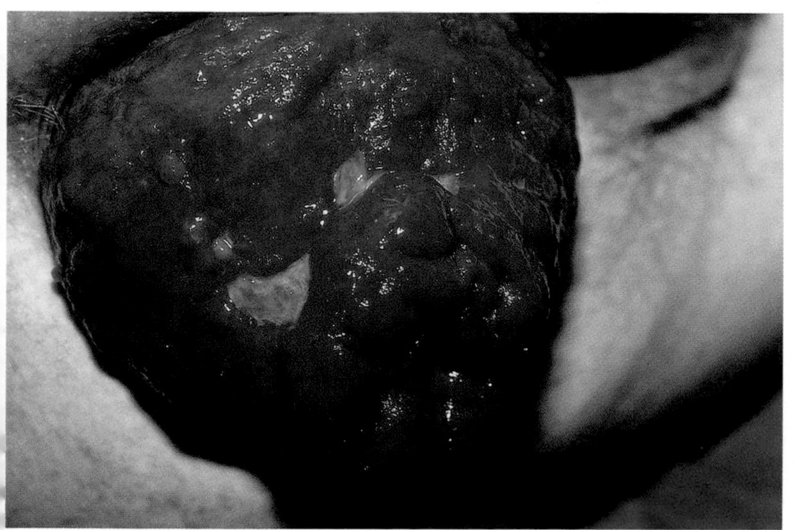

Fig. 124 Prolapsed rectum with associated ulceration.

51 Anal warts (condyloma acuminata)

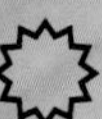

Aetiology

Warts in the perianal region have the same pathology and viral aetiology (human papilloma virus) as warts elsewhere but are usually transmitted by sexual activity.

Clinical features

Anal warts cause discomfort, pain, pruritus ani and difficulty with perianal hygiene. The warts are obvious externally (Fig. 125).

Management

In small numbers anal warts can be treated by topical application of podophyllin. More extensive cases may require treatment with diathermy or surgical excision (Figs 126, 127). Normal skin between the warts is carefully preserved to avoid delayed healing or the disastrous complication of anal stenosis. Repeat operations are frequently indicated. Referral to a genitourinary medical unit may be appropriate if other sexually transmitted diseases are suspected.

Prognosis

Anal warts are associated with an increased risk of squamous carcinoma.

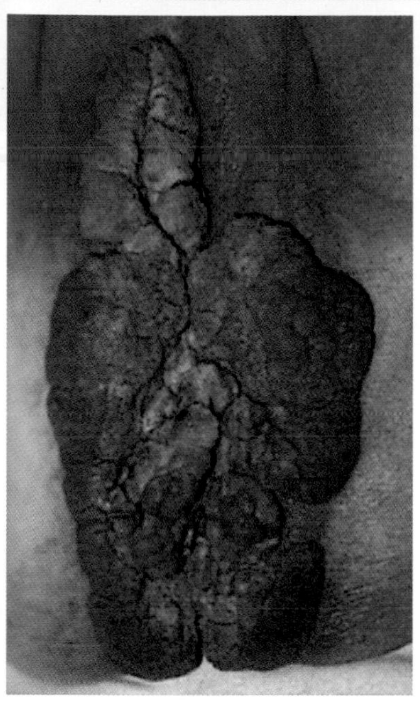

Fig. 125 Extensive anal warts that interfered with defaecation.

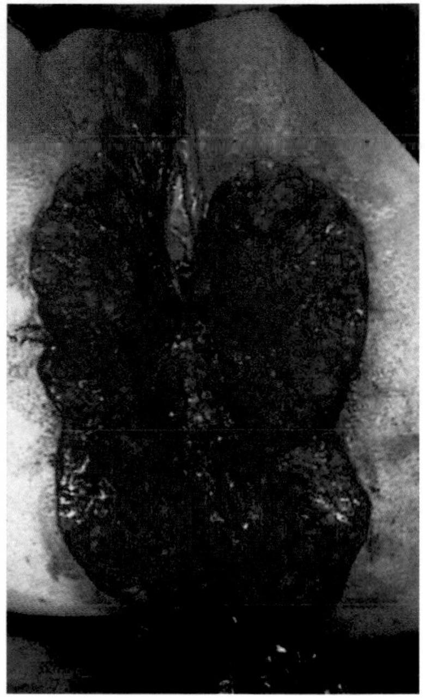

Fig. 126 The anal warts required radical excision.

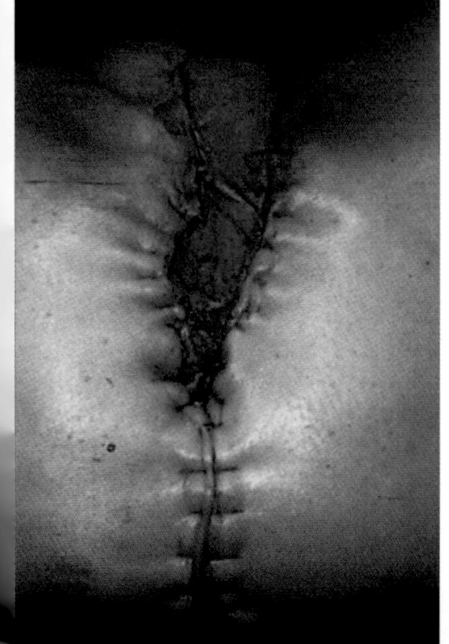

Fig. 127 The resulting defect was closed by mobilizing the adjacent skin flaps.

52 Anal cancer

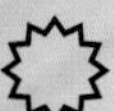

Incidence	Anal cancer is uncommon compared to colorectal cancer. The ratio of anal to colorectal cancer is approximately 1:25, although the incidence of anal cancer is increasing. Over 80% of anal cancer is squamous-cell carcinoma and approximately 10% of tumours are adenocarcinomas. Other rarer tumours include melanoma, lymphoma and sarcoma. Most patients with anal cancer present in the sixth and seventh decades.
Aetiology	The aetiology is not fully defined but population studies show there is an association between anal and cervical cancer. Anal warts are also a risk factor, as is anal intercourse.
Clinical features	Patients may present with anal pain, bleeding or discharge and pruritus ani. Advanced cases may present with faecal incontinence. Clinical examination may reveal an ulcerated lesion at the anal verge that is hard to palpation (Figs 128, 129). Examination under anaesthesia is necessary in almost all cases to allow tissue biopsy and sigmoidoscopy. Histological confirmation of the diagnosis is essential as treatment varies depending on the tissue of origin.
Management	Modern treatment of anal cancer is multidisciplinary. The current standard treatment for squamous-cell cancer is radiotherapy to the anal canal and inguinal lymph nodes combined with 5 fluorouracil and mitomycin C. Surgery may play a part in the management of advanced disease or in small tumours that can be completely excised.
Prognosis	The 5-year survival rate is approximately 60%.

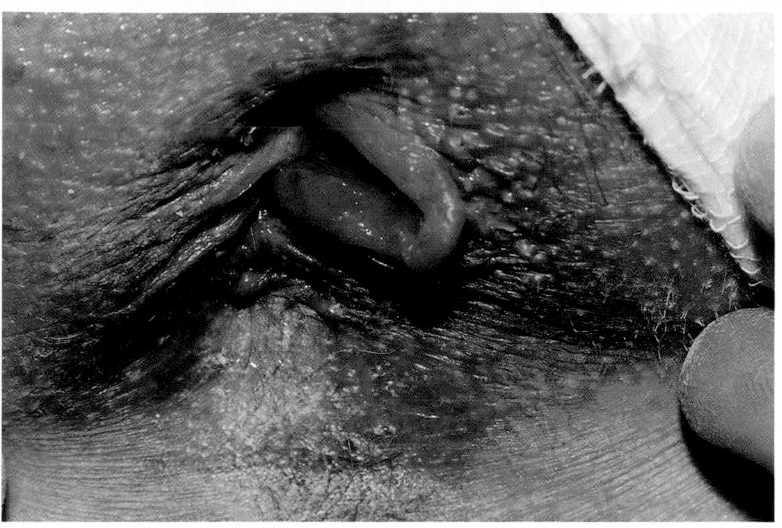

Fig. 128 Squamous-cell anal carcinoma.

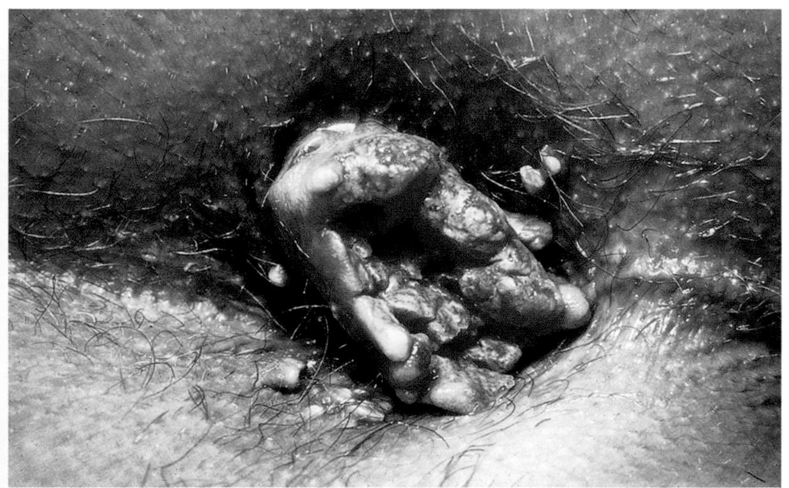

Fig. 129 Squamous-cell anal carcinoma.

53 Ileostomy

Definition

An ileostomy is a stoma in which the small bowel opens on to the anterior abdominal wall.

Classification

- End stoma
- Loop stoma
- Defunctioning stoma

Aetiology

An ileostomy may be employed as an adjunct to resectional surgery where the disease process prevents re-anastomosis, or as a temporary stoma to allow a distal anastomosis to heal, such as for a low colorectal or ileoanal anastomosis.

Management

An ileostomy is usually fashioned in the right iliac fossa (Figs 130–132). As the small bowel contents are fluid and contain active proteolytic enzymes, a spout is fashioned to enable the discharge from the ileostomy to be directed into an appliance preserving the surrounding skin. Ileostomies, unlike colostomies, discharge continuously and an appliance must be worn at all times.

Urostomy

If the urinary bladder is resected the ureters can be drained into an isolated segment of small bowel that is brought out as a spout (an ileal conduit) in a similar fashion to an ileostomy, to enable urine to discharge into an appliance.

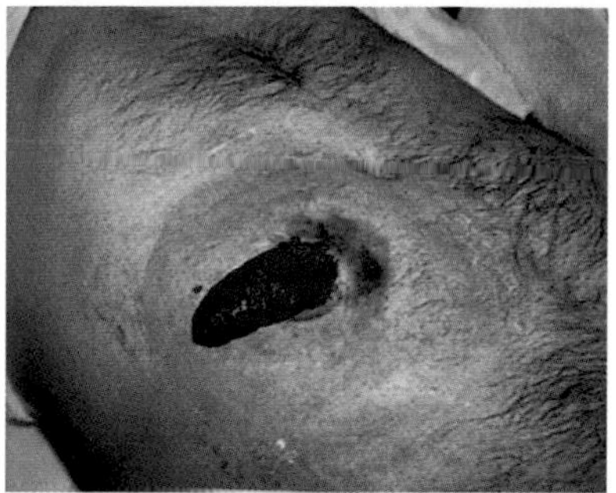

Fig. 130 Ileostomy sited in the right iliac fossa.

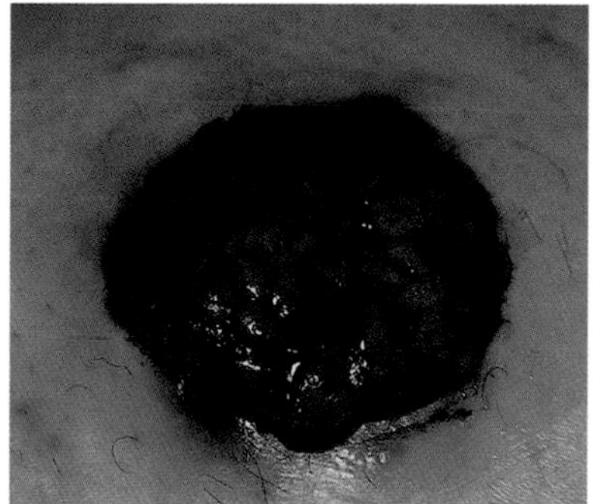

Fig. 131 Ileostomy affected by Crohn's disease.

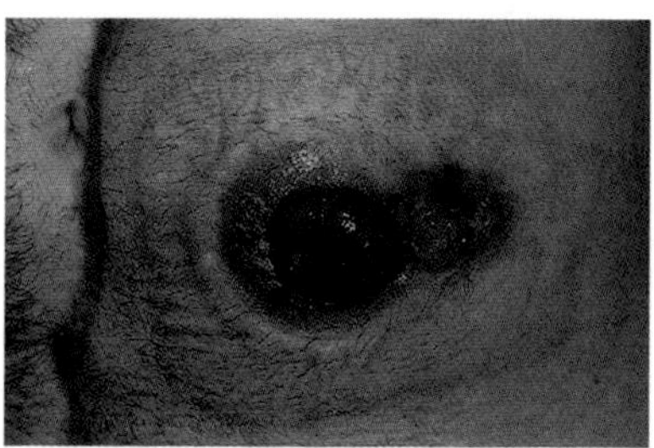

Fig. 132 Ileostomy with parastomal ulceration due to underlying Crohn's disease.

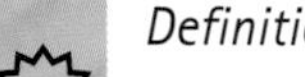

54 Colostomy

Definition

A colostomy is an opening of the colon on to skin (Fig. 134, 135).

Classification

- End colostomy – is fashioned during a Hartman's procedure and is an integral part of an abdominal perineal (AP) resection
- Loop colostomy – is used to divert faeces from a diseased anus/rectum, after difficult anastomotic surgery to promote healing without a faecal stream, or as a palliative procedure for pelvic cancer.

Management

Colostomies are usually fashioned in the left iliac fossa, although a transverse colostomy may rarely be undertaken in the upper abdomen. The discharge from a colostomy is solid or semi-solid and the bowel is joined flush to the skin without creating a spout.

Complications

- Ischemia due to strangulation
- Obstruction due to oedema or faecal impaction
- Skin erosion
- Prolapse of bowel
- Parastomal hernia
- Parastomal fistula
- Retraction of spout
- Stenosis of stomal orifice.

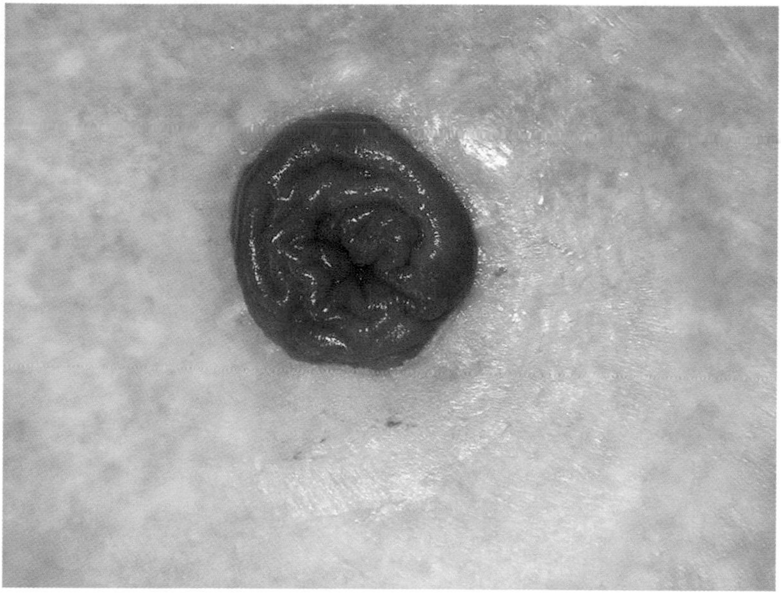

Fig. 133 Colostomy in a patient following abdominal–perineal resection.

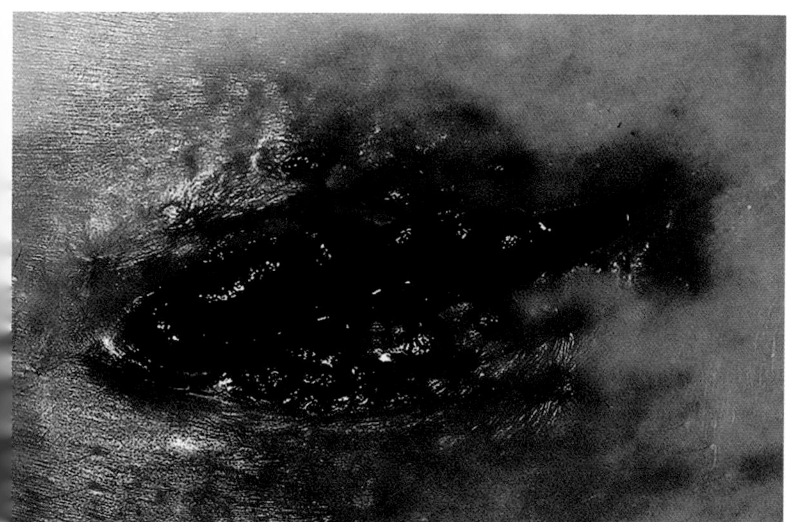

Fig. 134 Crohn's disease of colostomy.

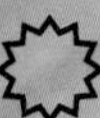

55 Aneurysmal arterial disease

Definition

An aneurysm is an abnormal localized dilatation of a blood vessel. Arterial aneurysms (Figs 135–138) are by far the most common.

Classification

Anatomical

- Localized (saccular)
- Diffuse (fusiform)

Pathological

- True (lined by all three layers of the normal arterial wall)
- False or pseudo- (formed in the adventitia or completely outside the wall of the vessel)

Aetiology

- Atherosclerosis
- Inflammation (approximately 10% of abdominal aortic aneurysms have an inflammatory element)
- Infection (certain organisms, notably *Salmonella* spp. and *Treponema pallidum*, have a particular ability to infect the aortic wall, causing a mycotic aneurysm)

Complications

Surgeons operate on aneurysms to prevent or manage complications such as rupture. Other complications include thrombosis and distal embolism. Less frequently, aneurysms cause external compression or stretching of surrounding structures.

Femoral aneurysm

Femoral aneurysms present as a pulsatile lump in the groin. True femoral aneurysms are uncommon but a false aneurysm in this area may follow femoral artery instrumentation.

Popliteal aneurysm

Popliteal aneurysms most often cause symptoms because of emboli (ischaemic toes) or thrombosis (ischaemic lower limb). Rupture is uncommon. The aneurysm presents as a pulsatile swelling behind the knee and is easily palpated. The differential diagnosis is a Baker's cyst. Popliteal aneurysms are commonly bilateral.

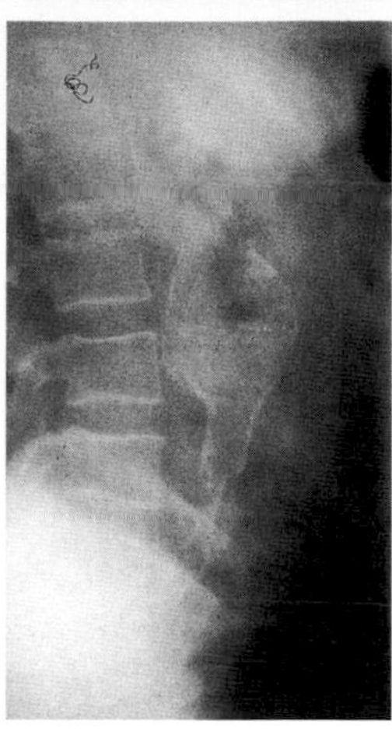

Fig. 135 Lateral abdominal X-ray demonstrating an abdominal aortic aneurysm.

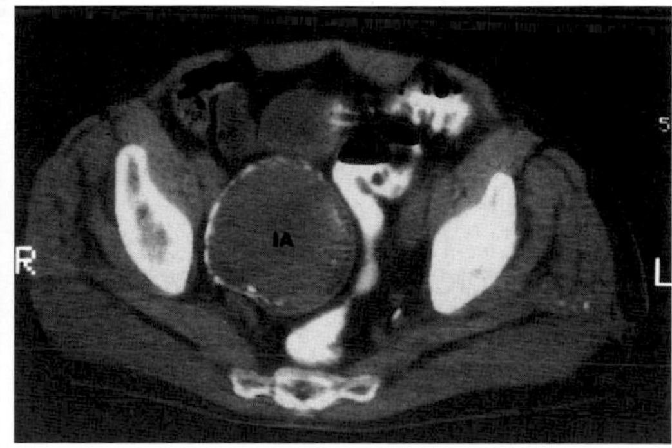

Fig. 136 CT scan demonstrating a large aortoiliac aneurysm.

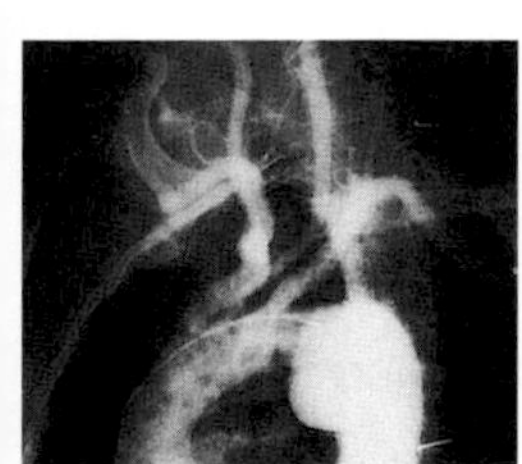

Fig. 137 Thoracic aortography demonstrating a thoracic aortic aneurysm.

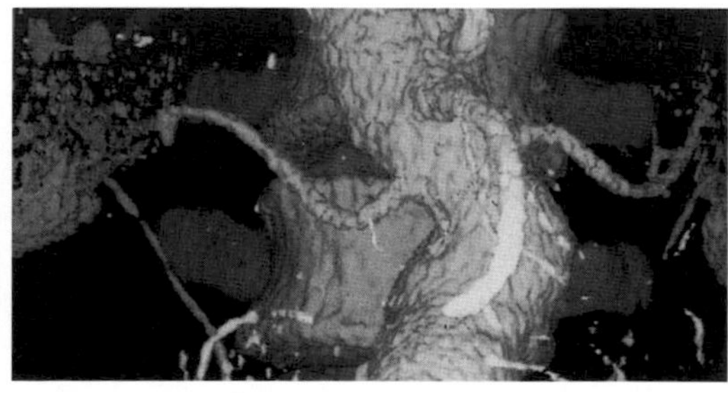

Fig. 138 Three-dimensional reconstruction from spiral CT scan showing an abdominal aortic aneurysm.

56 Abdominal aortic aneurysm

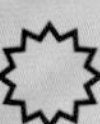

Incidence

An abdominal aortic aneurysm (AAA) is present in 5% of men aged over 60 years and accounts for 1% of deaths in this group. They are three times more common in men than woman. 70% of cases affect only the infrarenal segment of the aorta.

Clinical features

- Asymptomatic (30%) –may be detected incidentally on routine clinical examination, plain abdominal X-ray or by ultrasonography (Fig. 139)
- Symptomatic (20%) – may cause abdominal or back pain and may mimic renal colic with pain radiating from the back to the loin or groin
- Thrombotic emboli may migrate to the lower limbs causing acute lower limb ischaemia. Less commonly an AAA may undergo thrombotic occlusion
- Rupture (50%) – may rupture into the retroperitoneum or peritoneal cavity causing acute symptoms/or collapse (Fig. 140). Less commonly an AAA may rupture into the inferior vena cava leading to an aortocaval fistula (Fig. 141).

Management

Ultrasonography is the best investigation to establish the diagnosis and to ascertain the size of the aneurysm. Small aneurysms can be reassessed on a regular basis to see if they increase in size. Elective surgical repair of an AAA should be considered when it reaches 5.0 cm in diameter. All symptomatic AAA should be considered for repair as the likelihood of rupture is high. Open surgical repair of an AAA entails replacing the aneurysmal segment with a prosthetic graft. Some AAAs may be treated with a covered stent placed via a femoral arteriotomy under radiological guidance. At present only a proportion of AAAs are suitable for this technique and this is usually in the elective setting.

Prognosis

The 30-day mortality for elective repair of an asymptomatic AAA is 5–8%, for an emergency symptomatic AAA repair 10–20% and for a ruptured AAA approximately 50%. The long-term survival for patients who are discharged from hospital approaches that of the normal population.

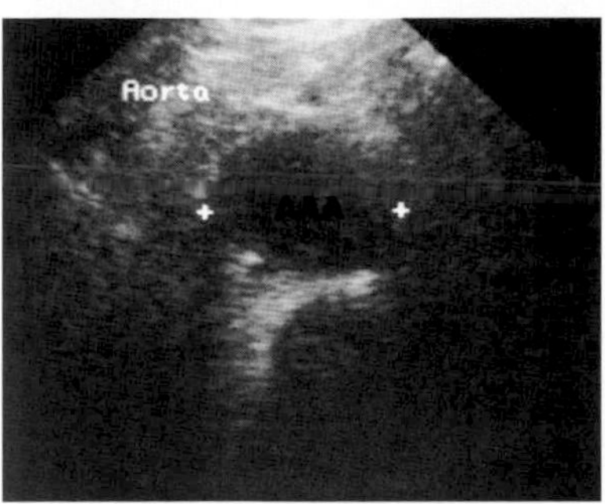

A

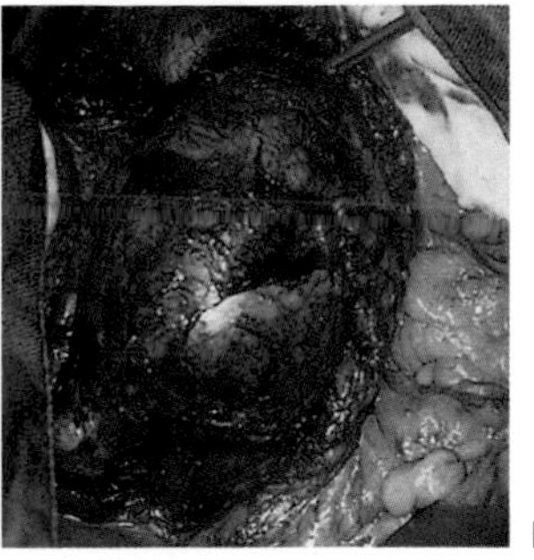

B

Fig. 139 **A.** Ultrasound scan of an abdominal aortic aneurysm. **B.** At operation the aneurysm is isolated and repair is undertaken by insertion of a synthetic graft.

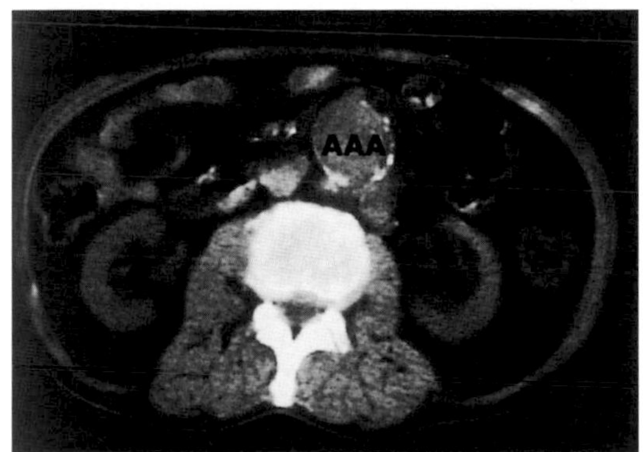

Fig. 140 CT scan confirming a ruptured abdominal aortic aneurysm.

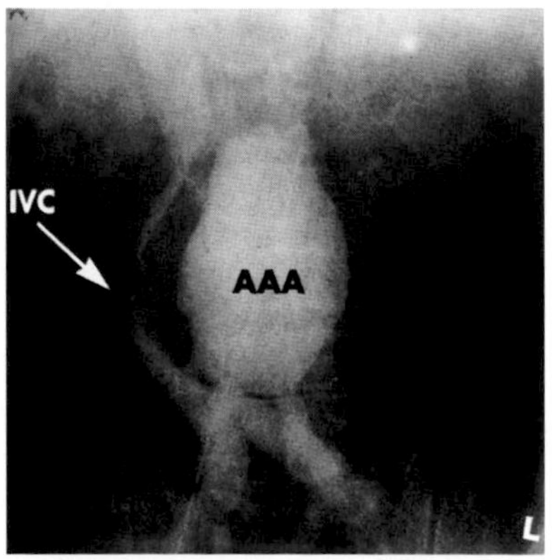

Fig. 141 Aortocaval fistula demonstrated by angiography.

57 Acute limb ischaemia

Aetiology

- Thrombosis (60%) – acute occlusion of a pre-existing stenotic arterial segment.
- Embolism (30%) – may arise from mural thrombus in the heart after myocardial infarction, from the left atrial appendix in atrial fibrillation, from the aorta or other major vessel that is aneurysmal or atherosclerotic, or rarely vegetations dislodge from a heart valve in endocarditis or rheumatic disease.
- Trauma (10%) – may be iatrogenic.

Clinical features

- Pain
- Pallor
- Pulseless
- Perishing cold
- Parasthesia
- Paralysis.

In acute ischaemia due to embolism (Fig. 143), onset is usually very sudden and a potential cause, such as atrial fibulation, may often be recognized. In cases due to acute thrombosis, there may be a history of intermittent claudication and pulses/pressures in the contralateral limb may be reduced (Fig. 142).

Management

Acute limb ischaemia is the most common vascular emergency and all patients should be discussed immediately with a vascular surgeon. An intravenous bolus of heparin should be administered to limit propagation of thrombus. Subsequent management depends on whether the limb is deemed non-viable, threatened or non-threatened. If the limb is non-viable a decision must be taken as to whether it is appropriate to consider amputation or palliation. Features of a threatened ischaemic limb include loss of sensation, loss of active movement and pain on passive movement when the calf muscles are squeezed. In these circumstances an urgent embolectomy or thrombectomy should be undertaken. A period of medical optimization on heparin therapy may lead to spontaneous improvement in a non-threatened limb. Thrombolysis may be attempted in these circumstances.

Complications

- Reperfusion injury – this can lead to acute respiratory distress syndrome (ARDS), endotoxaemia, acute tubular necrosis and multiple organ failure
- Compartment syndrome – this can lead to muscle necrosis despite adequate arterial inflow; fasciotomy should be performed if this complication is suspected (Fig. 144).

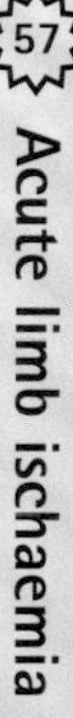

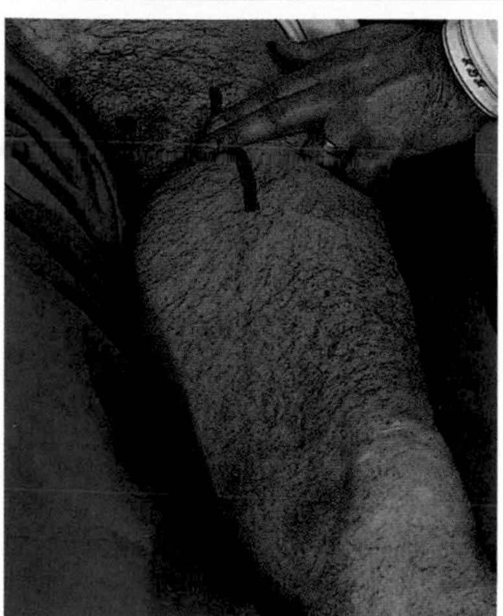

Fig. 142 Palpation of the femoral artery. Pulses should be compared on either side.

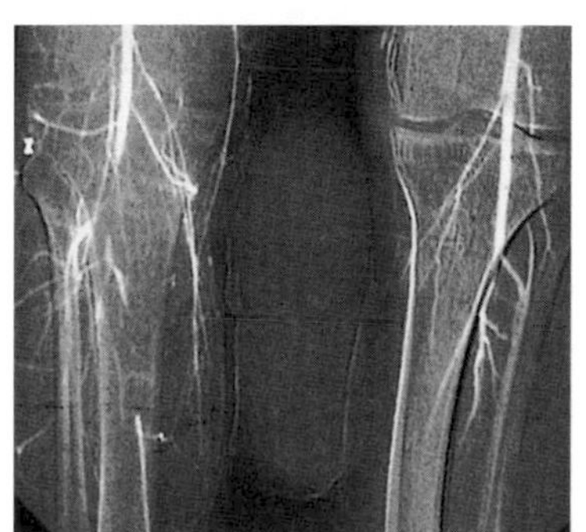

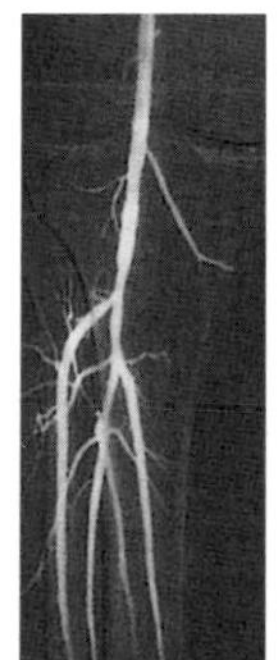

A B

Fig. 143 **A.** Acute lower limb ischaemia caused by a popliteal embolus. **B.** Successful popliteal embolectomy was confirmed by on-table check angiography.

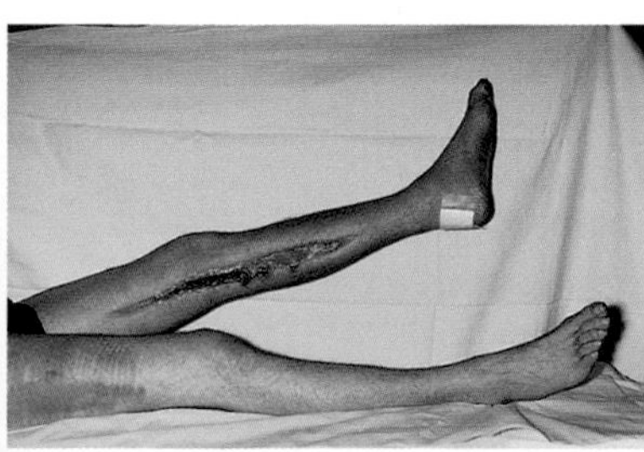

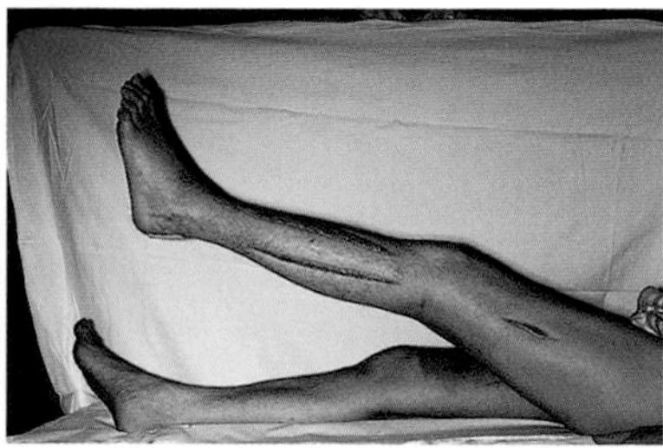

A B

Fig. 144 A&B Healing fasciotomy wounds after management of compartment syndrome. Note that the three compartments of the left lower limb have been previously decompressed.

58 Chronic limb ischaemia (1)

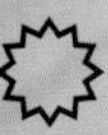

Intermittent claudication

Definition

Intermittent claudication is a muscular pain brought on by exercise and relieved by rest.

Incidence

Intermittent claudication is the mildness manifestation of chronic lower limb ischaemia and affects approximately 5% of men over 60 years of age. It is usually the consequence of atherosclerotic narrowing or occlusion of the superficial femoral artery in the thigh (Figs 145, 146).

Clinical features

Intermittent claudication usually causes pain in the muscles of the calf, however if the iliac arteries are affected then the pain may also be felt in the thigh or buttock (Leriche's syndrome). The pain comes on after a reasonably constant 'claudication distance' and subsides rapidly and completely on cessation of walking. Pulses are usually diminished or absent below the femoral level (Figs 147, 148), but if they are present, exercise causes them to disappear.

Differential diagnosis

- Pain from the back, hip or knee joint due to osteoarthritis
- Venous outflow obstruction (venous claudication)
- Neurogenic pain

Management

Patients should be advised to stop smoking. They should be screened and treated for correctable risk factors such as diabetes and hyperlipidaemia. Patients should be told to exercise regularly to the point of pain in order to develop collateral circulation. Percutaneous transluminal angioplasty has not been shown to confer any additional long-term benefit over best medical therapy. Few patients with intermittent claudication require vascular reconstructive surgery.

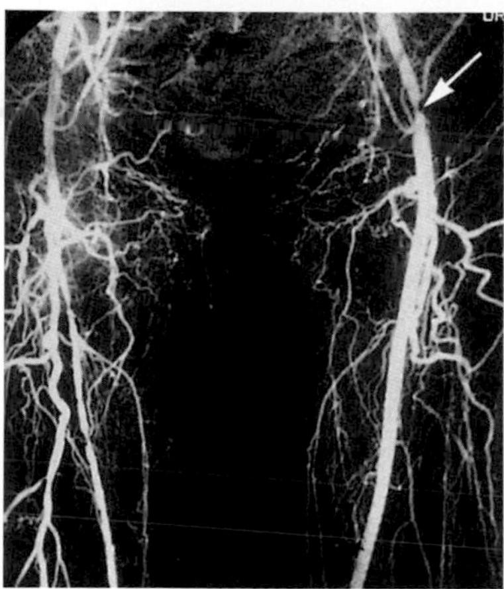

Fig. 145 Common femoral artery stenosis.

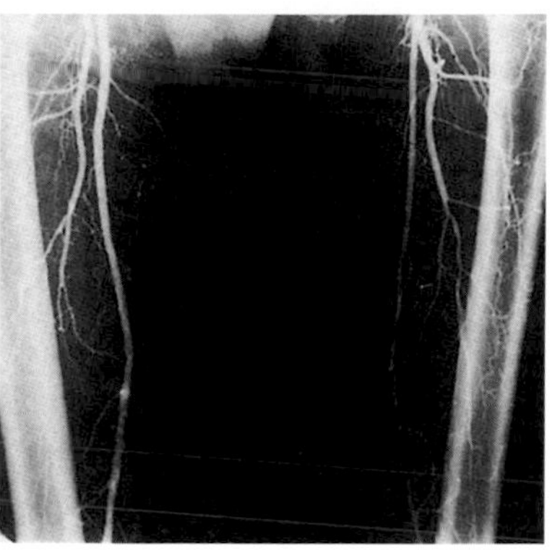

Fig. 146 Superficial femoral artery occlusion.

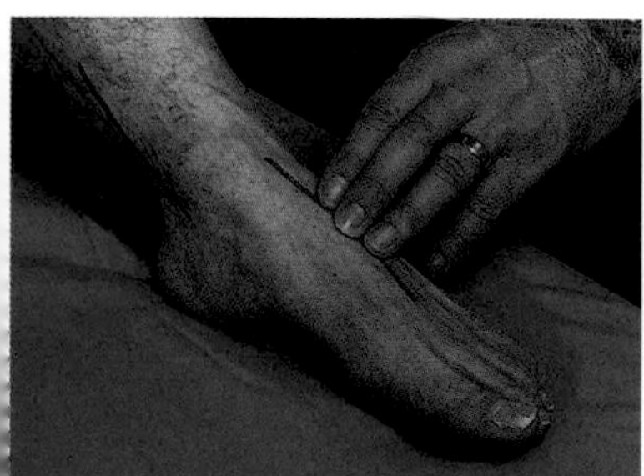

Fig. 147 Palpation of the dorsalis pedis artery.

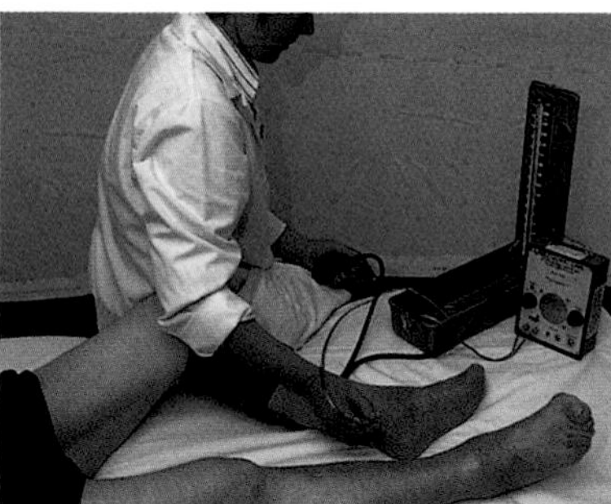

Fig. 148 A Doppler ultrasound probe can be used to obtain the blood pressure at which the signal in the artery disappears to give the perfusion pressure. The ankle brachial pressure index (ABPI) gives an indication of the perfusion to the lower limb.

59 Chronic limb ischaemia (2)

Critical limb ischaemia

Definition

Critical limb ischaemia is defined as rest pain that requires strong analgesia for a period of 2 weeks or more, and tissue loss in association with an ankle pressure of less than 50 mmHg (European consensus document). The inference is that, without intervention, a patient with critical limb ischaemia will come to major amputation within weeks or months.

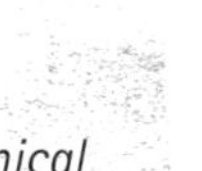

Clinical features

Rest pain is indicative of severe ischaemia. It is usually felt in the forefoot and typically the pain is worst at night, obliging the patient to hang the foot out of bed, walk about or sleep sitting upright in a chair to lessen the pain. The reasons for night and rest pain are an increased metabolic rate in the foot under the warm bedclothes, reduced cardiac output and blood pressure during sleep, and loss of the beneficial effect of gravity.

Classical signs of chronic ischaemia include slow capillary refill and pallor on elevating the limb. Marked rubor and cyanosis in a dependent foot following elevation of the limb is known as a positive Buerger's test (Fig. 149).

Management

Medical measures such as treatment of heart failure, intercurrent infection, anaemia and diabetes should be optimized; however, invasive intervention is usually required. Percutaneous transluminal balloon angioplasty may be helpful, but many patients require arterial surgical reconstruction. Amputation is a last resort.

Prognosis

Surgical reconstruction is associated with a mortality rate of 1–5%. In hospital mortality for patients requiring major limb amputation is approximately 10–20%.

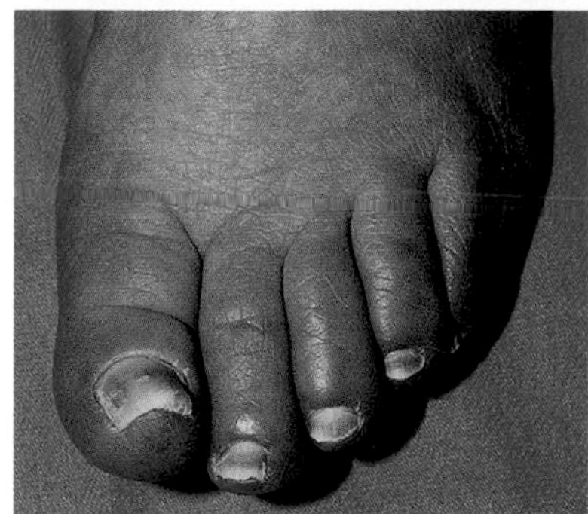

Fig. 149 The combination of pallor on elevation and dependent rubor is known as Buerger's sign and is a feature of critical limb ischaemia.

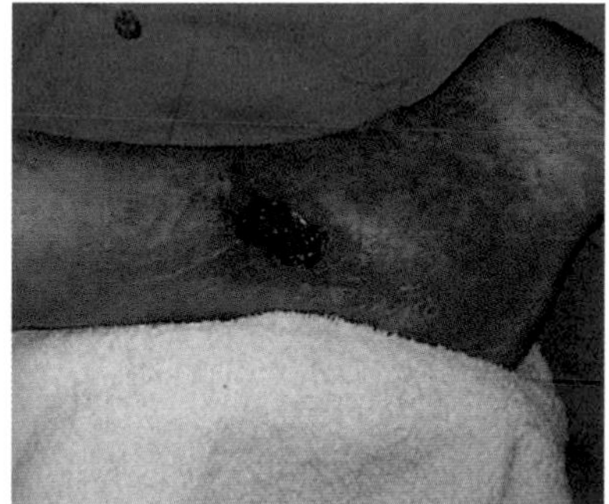

Fig. 150 Ischaemic foot ulcer.

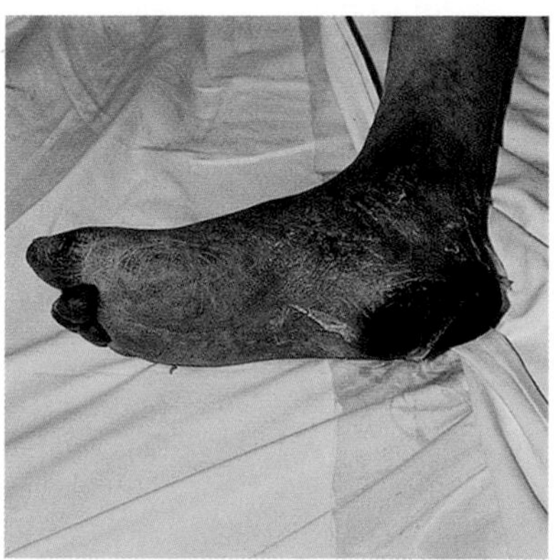

Fig. 151 Necrotic heel in a patient with critical limb ischaemia.

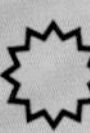

60 Gangrene

Definition

Gangrene is the presence of dead tissue and is the end stage of peripheral vascular disease (Fig. 152).

Classification

- Dry gangrene – non-infected
- Wet gangrene – infected.

Clinical features

Dry gangrene occurs when dead tissue mummifies without infection. The toes are most commonly infected and the result is a dry black digit with a sharp line of demarcation with healthy living tissue (Fig. 153).

If the necrotic area becomes infected, the tissue becomes boggy and the gangrene spreads proximally (Fig. 154). Clostridia are the usual causal organisms and the tissue becomes foul-smelling. The dead tissue is in continuity with living tissue and as a result toxins reach the circulation and make the patient systemically unwell.

Management

Dry gangrene usually results in the affected area separating from the healthy tissue spontaneously; this is known as auto-amputation. Wet gangrene requires urgent treatment with the combination of revascularization and debridement or amputation (Fig. 155).

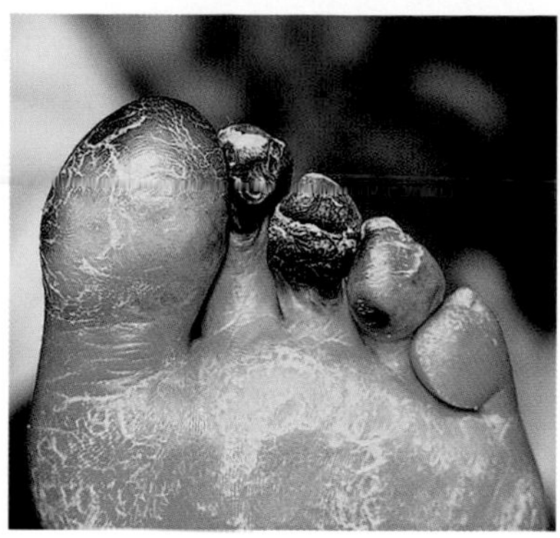

Fig. 152 Gangrene is the end-stage of peripheral vascular disease.

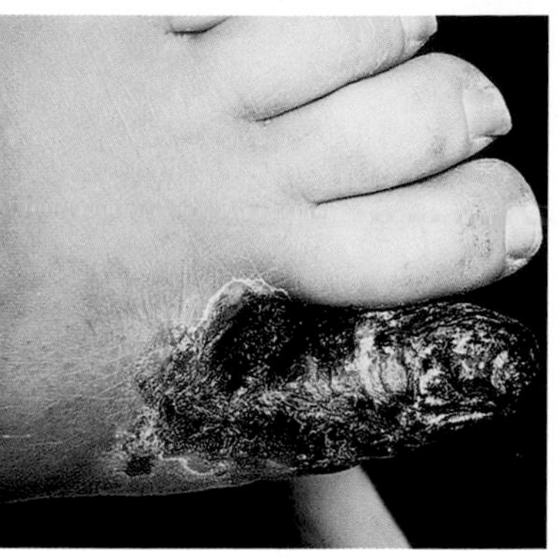

Fig. 153 Dry gangrene of the left great toe.

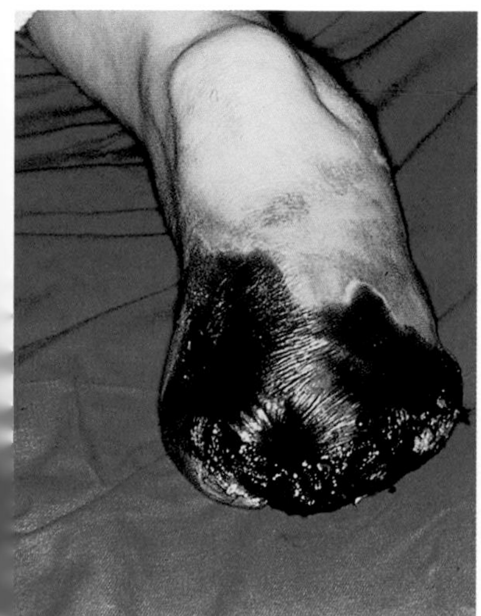

Fig. 154 Wet gangrene affecting the stump of a below knee amputation.

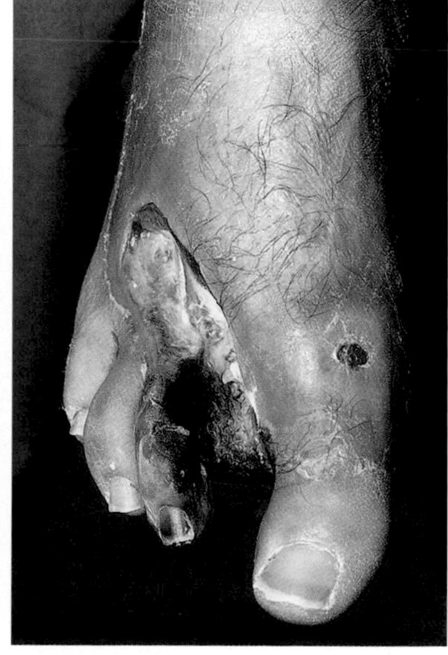

Fig. 155 Ray amputation of right second toe.

61 The diabetic foot

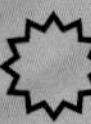

Incidence	• Diabetic foot problems account for 12% of all medical hospital admissions • 80% of patients with diabetic foot problems have type 2 diabetes • Foot problems are responsible for approximately half of the time spent in hospital by diabetic patients
Aetiology	Diabetic patients are prone to serious ulceration and infection of the feet. Several factors may contribute to diabetic foot problems. • Atherosclerosis – particularly affecting smaller arteries of the lower limb and feet (Fig. 156) • Sensory neuropathy – reduces sensation so injury occurs unnoticed • Autonomic neuropathy – causes a lack of sweating, resulting in dry, fissured skin, which permits entry of bacteria • Motor neuropathy – results in wasting and weakness of the small muscles of the feet causing deformities with pressure points and Charcot's joints
Clinical features	Foot complications of diabetic neuropathy present as: • Painless, deeply penetrating ulcers – predominantly under the metatarsal heads • Infection, which may spread through plantar spaces and along the tendon sheaths and result in deep sinuses • Chronic ulceration of pressure points and at sites of minor injury • Extensive spreading skin necrosis • Painless necrosis of individual toes.
Management	The principles of management of diabetic foot complications are: • Control of infection – this may include intravenous antibiotics and drainage of pus • Removal of necrotic tissue – by a desloughing procedure or amputation • Attention to blood glucose control • If there is ischaemia, revascularization should be considered.
Prognosis	Recurrent problems are frequently encountered and high risk patients should be regularly seen by chiropody services. Careful attention should be given to footwear to correct abnormal pressure patterns.

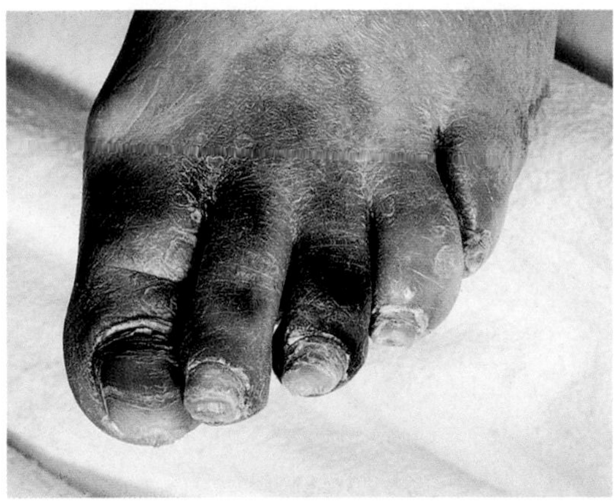

Fig. 156 Patient with small-vessel disease secondary to diabetes.

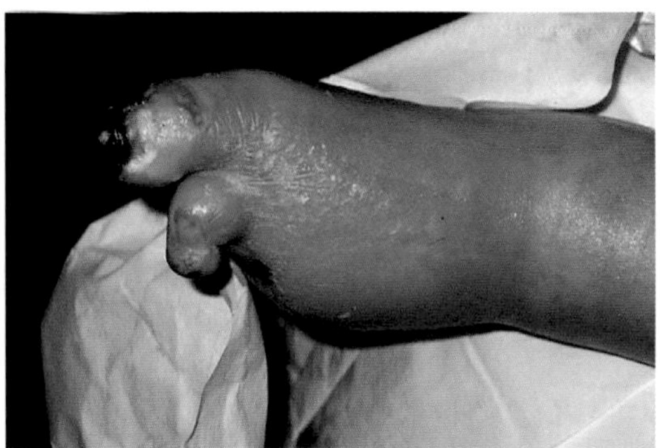

Fig. 157 Diabetic foot with previous amputation of digits.

62 Raynaud's phenomenon

Definition

Episodic digital (fingers or toes) vasospasm in the absence of an identifiable associated vascular disorder. Usually precipitated by exposure to cold.

Incidence

Raynaud's phenomenon is 10 times commoner in women than men. It affects 5–10% of females and there may be an associated family history.

Clinical features

There are three phases:

- Pallor – because of vasospasm of digital arteries (Fig. 158)
- Cyanosis – due to the presence of deoxygenated blood
- Rubor (redness) – due to reactive hyperaemia upon restoration of blood flow.

Management

Patients should be advised to stop smoking and to avoid exposure to cold. Numerous drugs have been tried with inconsistent results. The calcium channel blocker nifedipine is the most commonly prescribed medication but it may cause side effects. Sympathectomy may be beneficial for lower limb vasospasm but it is associated with poor long-term results in the hand.

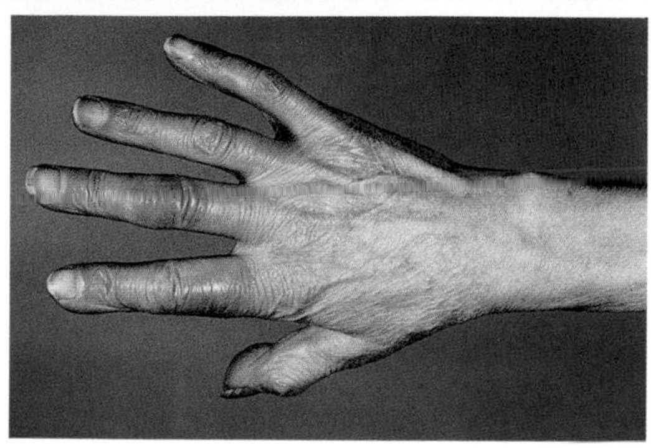
Fig. 158 In its mildest form, Raynaud's phenomenon causes white, numb and painful fingers in cold conditions.

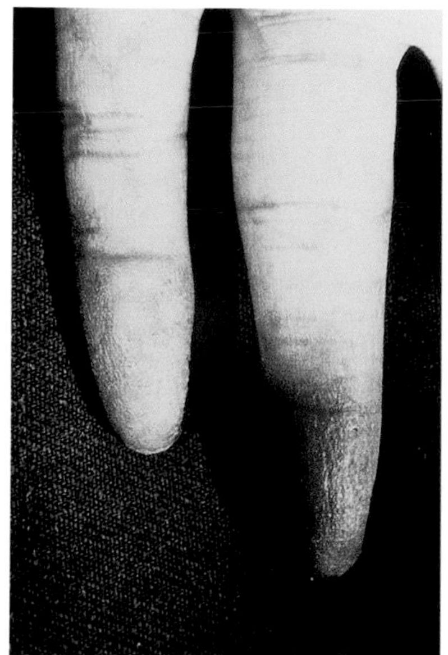
Fig. 159 Raynaud's phenomenon may cause fingertip necrosis.

63 Varicose veins

Definition

A vein is said to be varicose when its normal anatomy is distorted by dilatation and tortuosity.

Incidence

Approximately 20% of the adult population has varicose veins. The prevalence increases markedly with age and they are an almost universal finding in individuals over the age of 60 years.

Classification

- Primary – there is deep to superficial incompetence only, with no obvious underlying cause
- Secondary – varicosities develop because of some other cause, e.g. obstruction or thromboinflammatory destruction of valves in both the communicating and deep veins

Clinical features

Most varicose veins cause no symptoms and often the indication for seeking medical attention is because of the cosmetic appearance. Symptoms include heaviness, aching and ankle swelling.

The clinical appearance of varicose veins is of widened, elongated, tortuous veins that become more obvious on standing (Fig. 160). The distribution is usually in the territory of the long saphenous vein or the short saphenous vein.

Complications

Only a small proportion of patients with varicose veins develop the complications of chronic venous insufficiency – e.g. leg ulcers (Fig. 161), haemorrhage or thrombophlebitis.

Management

- Conservative treatment – elastic compression stockings, weight reduction, regular exercise and avoidance of prolonged standing
- Injection sclerotherapy – particularly suitable for small below-knee varicosities or for recurrent varicosities after surgery.
- Surgery – the saphenofemoral junction is ligated flush with the femoral vein, the long saphenous vein in the thigh may be stripped from the groin to the knee and the remaining varicosities are then avulsed through multiple tiny incisions.

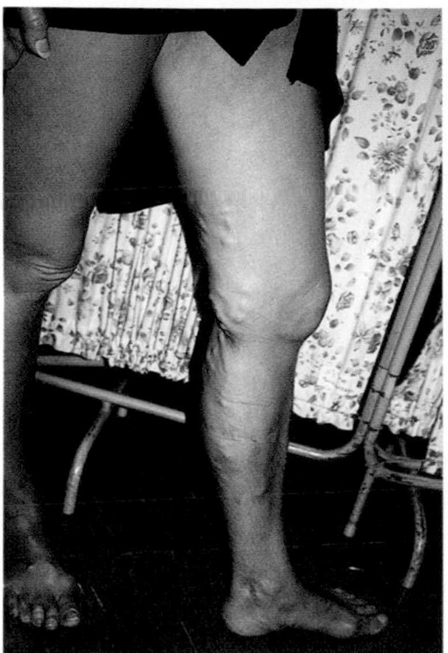

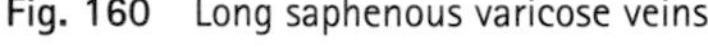

Fig. 160 Long saphenous varicose veins.

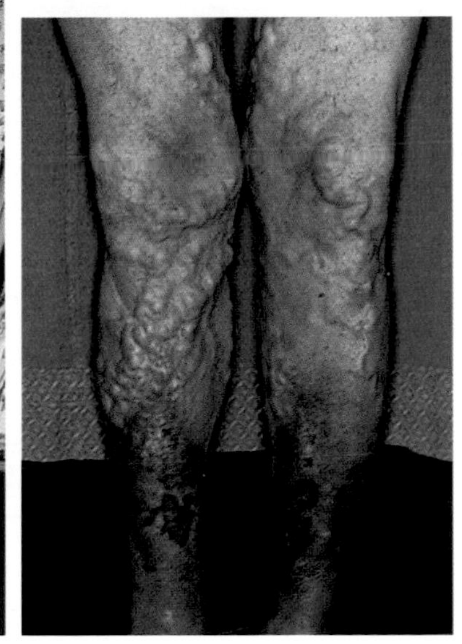

Fig. 161 Gross bilateral varicose veins with associated ulceration.

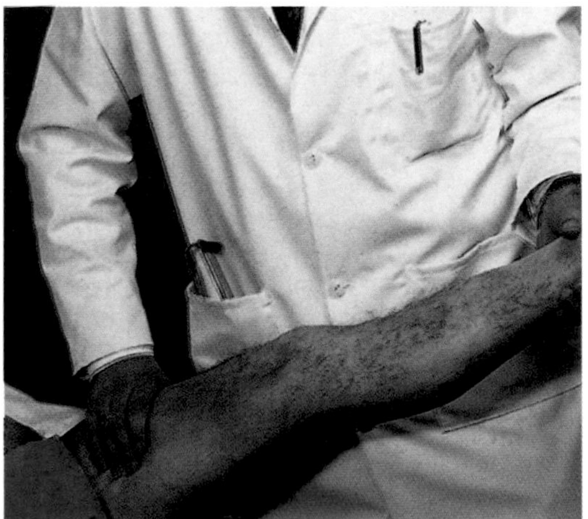

Fig. 162 Trendelenburg test of saphenofemoral incompetence.

64 Chronic venous insufficiency

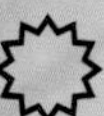

Definition

Chronic venous insufficiency may be defined as the presence of irreversible skin damage in the lower leg as a result of sustained venous hypertension.

Incidence

Chronic venous insufficiency affects 5–10% of the adult population. Chronic venous ulceration, the end result of chronic venous insufficiency, affects 2–3% of people over the age of 65. The female to male ratio is 3:1.

Aetiology

The two principal causes are long-standing varicose veins or previous venous obstruction due to deep venous thrombosis (DVT).

Clinical features

There may or may not be a history of previous DVT. Chronic venous hypertension in the skin results in lipodermatosclerosis (Fig. 163), pigmentation and eczematous change. Oedema is common but eventually fibrosis may produce scarred tissue around the ankle with oedema above.

Venous ulceration may be precipitated by minor trauma. It often occurs in an area of florid lipodermatosclerosis although sometimes there is little surrounding skin change. The most common site is over the medial or lateral malleolus and around the 'gaiter' area.

Superficial thrombophlebitis presents as a painful tender reddened area of skin overlying lower limb veins.

Management

It is important to establish whether or not there is deep vein occlusion. Patients with leg ulcers often require prolonged intensive treatment with compression stockings (Fig. 164). The 'four layer bandage' is a popular system. Surgical intervention may be required to correct superficial venous reflux, to disrupt medial calf perforators (Figs 165, 166) and to apply split-skin grafting to speed up ulcer healing.

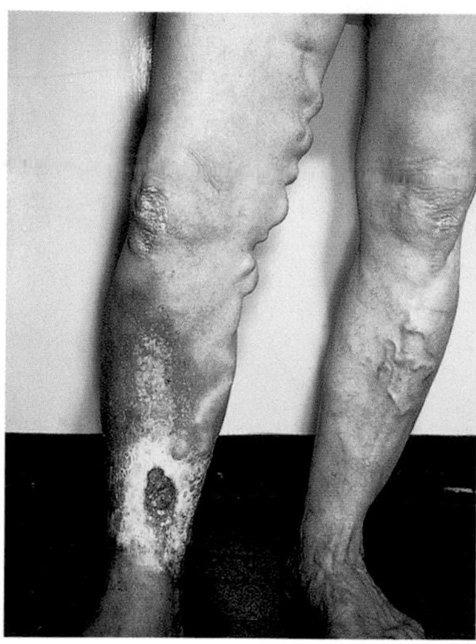

Fig. 163 Varicose ulceration with lipodermatosclerosis.

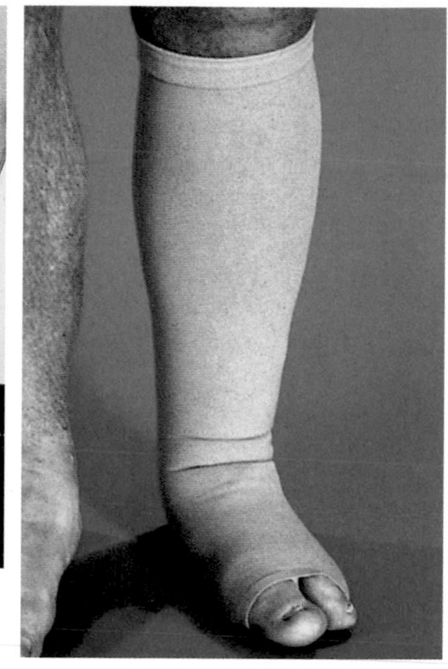

Fig. 164 Compression bandaging.

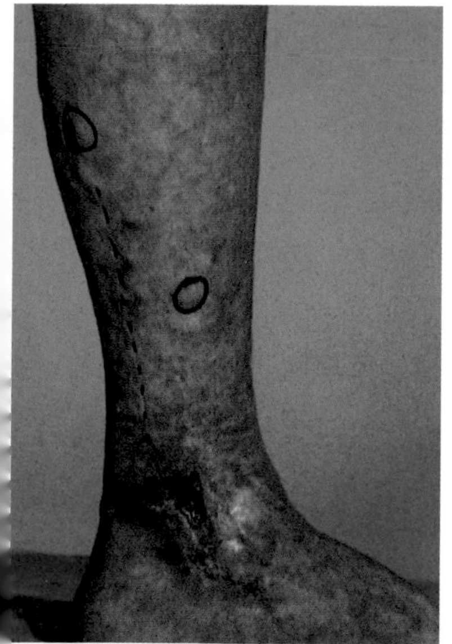

Fig. 165 Varicose ulcer with calf perforators shown.

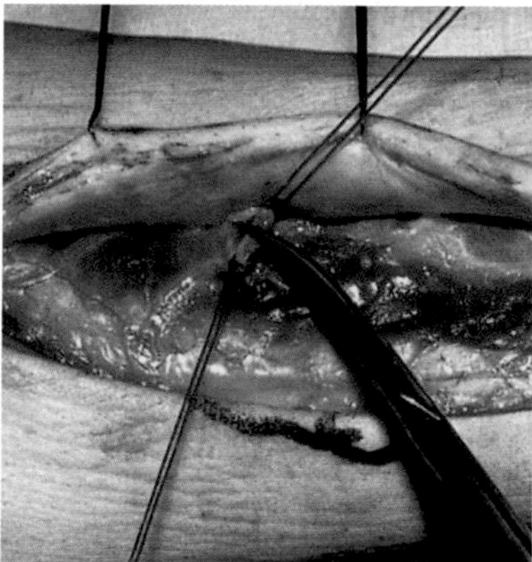

Fig. 166 Ligation of calf perforators at open surgery. A more recent innovation is endoscopic subfascial ligation.

65 Deep venous thrombosis

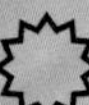

Aetiology

Deep venous thrombosis (DVT) usually involves the deep veins of the lower limb. Three factors are traditionally associated with development of a DVT – venous stasis, intimal damage and hypercoagulability of the blood (Virchow's triad). Many of the recognized clinical risk factors for DVT relate to venous stasis, e.g. post surgery, immobility, obesity and pregnancy. Hypercoagulable states include antithrombin III, protein C/protein S deficiency and malignancy.

Clinical features

Many DVTs are asymptomatic. However the principal symptoms are calf pain and swelling (Figs 167, 168). Physical signs include calf tenderness, oedema of the lower limb, distension of superficial veins and on occasion redness of the lower leg. Homans' sign (pain in the calf muscles on forced dorsiflexion of the ankle) should be abandoned.

Management

Colour duplex ultrasonography has largely replaced venography (Fig. 169) in the diagnosis of DVT. It is important to obtain an accurate diagnosis before treatment is instituted. However if the clinical suspicion of a DVT is high and there is no contraindication to heparinization, then the potential benefits of treatment may outweigh the risks. An uncomplicated DVT can now initially be treated with low-molecular-weight heparin injections. A continuous intravenous infusion of heparin is an alternative early treatment option. Most patients then require 6 months of oral anticoagulation. Surgical thrombectomy is rarely undertaken nowadays. A caval filter can be inserted if it is felt thrombi are passing to the lungs despite adequate anticoagulation, or if anticoagulation is contraindicated or has been discontinued because of a complication of therapy. Filters are usually inserted percutaneously under local anaesthesia by interventional radiologists via the jugular or femoral veins.

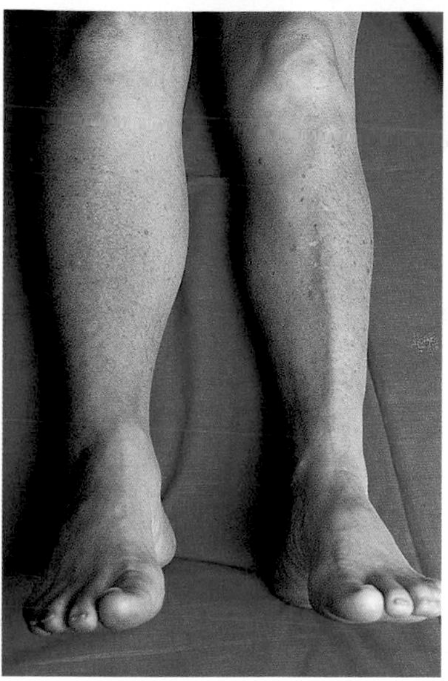

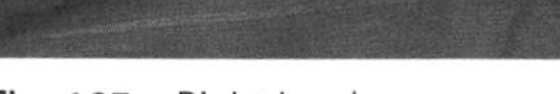

Fig. 167 Right leg deep venous thrombosis.

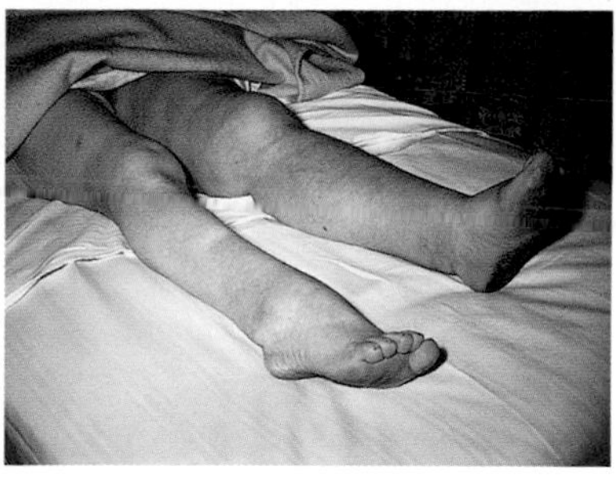

Fig. 168 Deep venous thrombosis of the left lower limb.

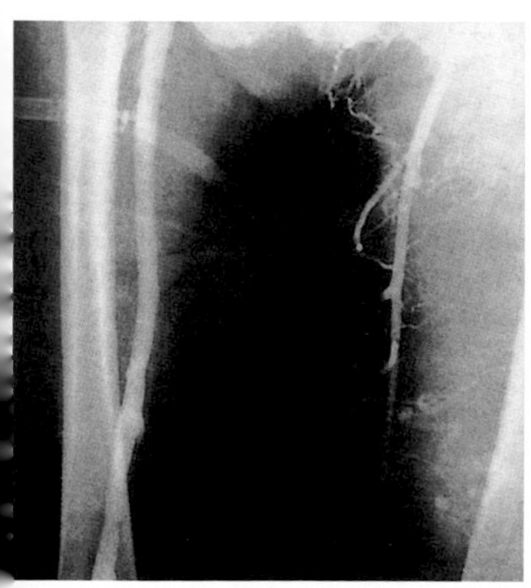

A

B

Fig. 169 A&B Bilateral ascending venogram showing occlusion of the left superficial femoral vein (A) and the iliac system with a tongue of thrombus lying within the inferior vena cava (B).

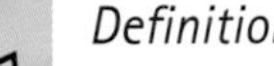

66 Lymphoedema

Definition

Lymphoedema is a swelling that results from an increased quantity of fluid in the interstitial spaces of soft tissue because of failure of function of the lymphatic drainage system.

Classification

- Primary – it is often a familial condition caused by a developmental failure (Fig. 170)
- Secondary – develops when the lymphatic system is obstructed by tumour, recurrent infection or infestation (filariasis) or obliterated by surgery or radiotherapy (Fig. 171).

Clinical features

The classical appearance is of a painless swelling of the limb. Initially this may be postural only but with time the oedema becomes persistent and associated with tissue fibrosis giving the classical 'non-pitting' oedema. Lymphoedema nearly always commences distally and extends proximally. Lymphoedema is essentially a clinical diagnosis and most patients do not require investigation.

Management

The principal of initial management is elevation of the swollen limb. Various forms of massage are effective at reducing oedema. Intermittent pneumatic compression devices are also useful. The mainstay of therapy is graduated compression hosiery. Diuretics are of no value and are more likely to cause troublesome side effects. Only a minority of patients will benefit from surgery and this is rarely performed.

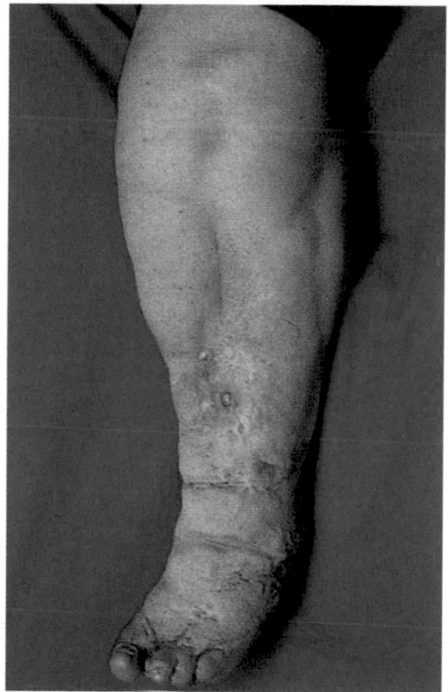

Fig. 170 Primary lymphoedema.

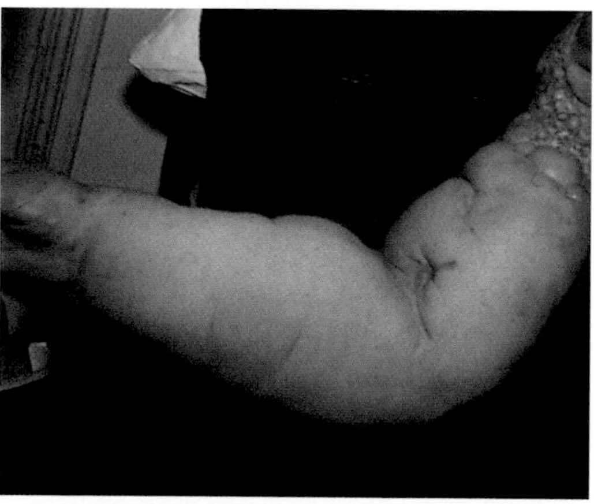

Fig. 171 Secondary lymphoedema due to axillary node involvement from a primary breast carcinoma.

Questions

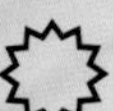

1. This elderly man presented with a longstanding abnormality affecting his nose.

a. What is the diagnosis and who typically develops this type of skin lesion?
b. Where is this lesion most commonly situated?
c. What is the mode of spread of this tumour?
d. What is the standard treatment?

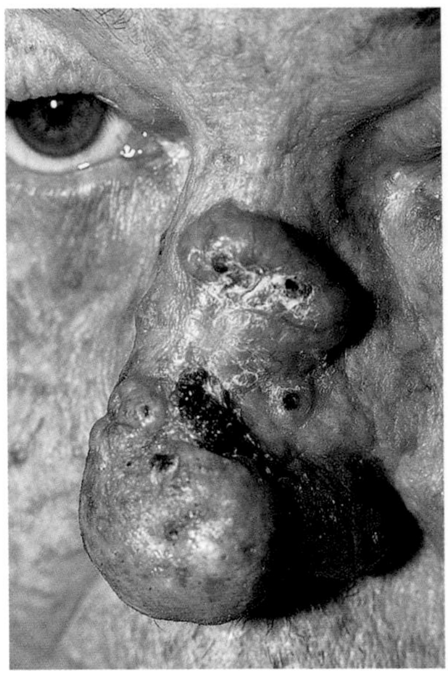

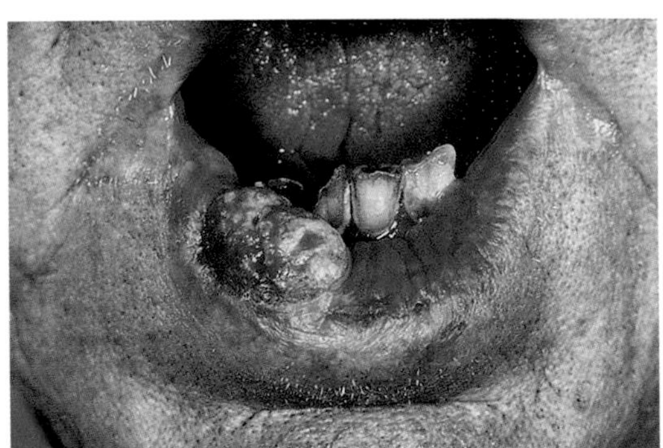

2. This lesion is on the lower lip of an elderly gentleman.

a. What is the likely diagnosis?
b. What is the main aetiological factor?
c. What is the treatment of choice?

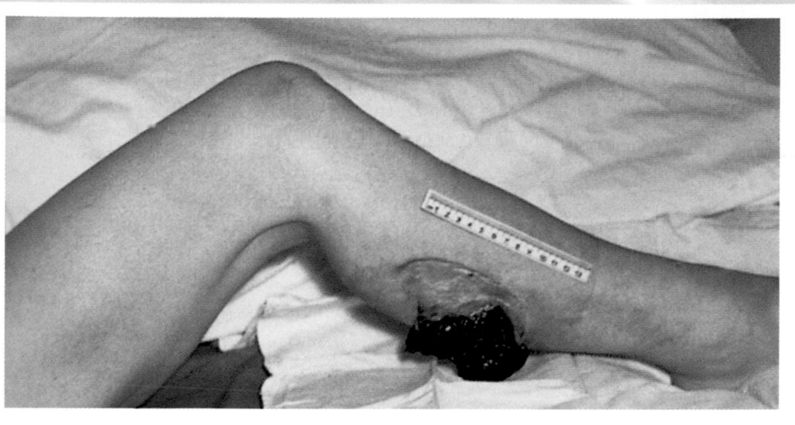

3. This lesion is on the right leg of a female patient

a. What is the lesion?
b. What clinical patterns of this lesion are described?
c. What is the management of such a lesion?
d. What is the prognosis for patients with this lesion?

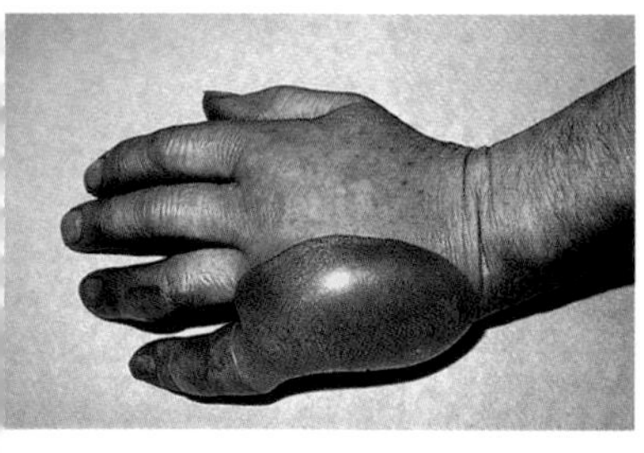

A

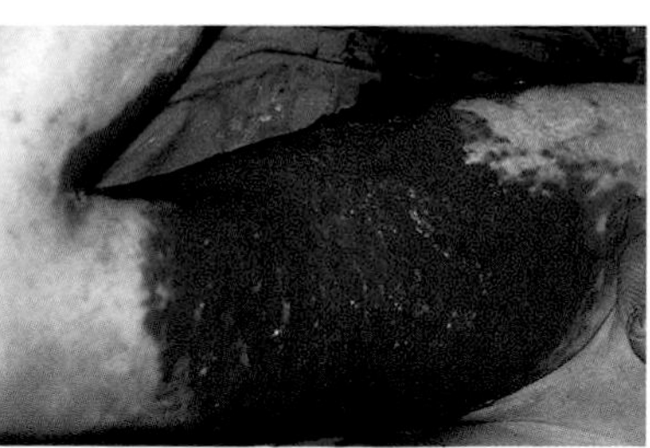

B

4. The two figures show the effects of a thermal injury.

a. What is the difference in classification of the two burn injuries?
b. How is the healing pattern different between a superficial and deep partial thickness burn?
c. What are the immediate management priorities in a patient with burn injury to the head and neck region?
d. What patients with thermal injuries are at greatest risk of burn shock?
e. What measures can be taken to reduce the development of disfiguring scar tissue and contractures?

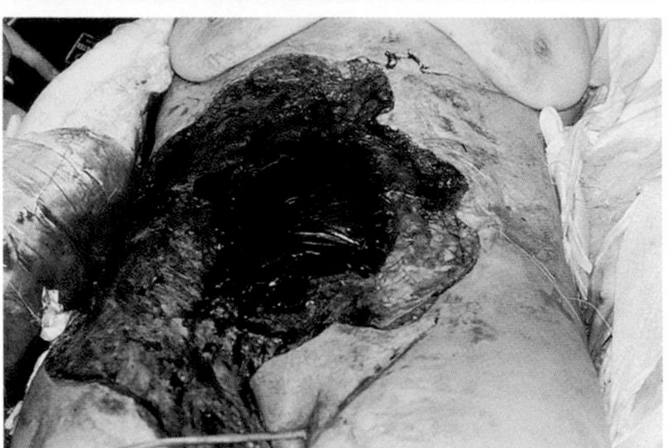

5. This patient required extensive debridement of the anterior abdominal wall.

a. What is the likely diagnosis?
b. What are the likely causative organisms?
c. What are the priorities in management?

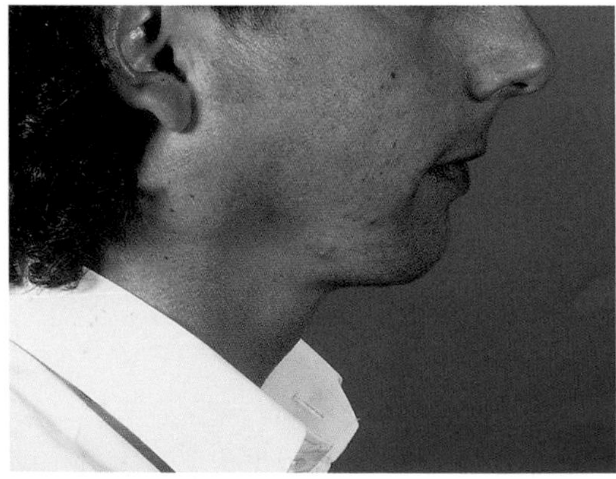

6. This patient noted a firm swelling over the angle of his jaw.

a. What is the likely diagnosis?
b. How does this tumour classically present?
c. How should such a lump be managed?
d. What is the most significant complication of parotidectomy?

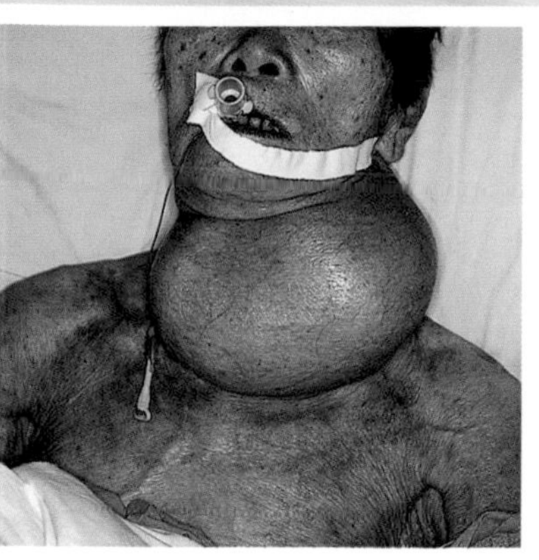

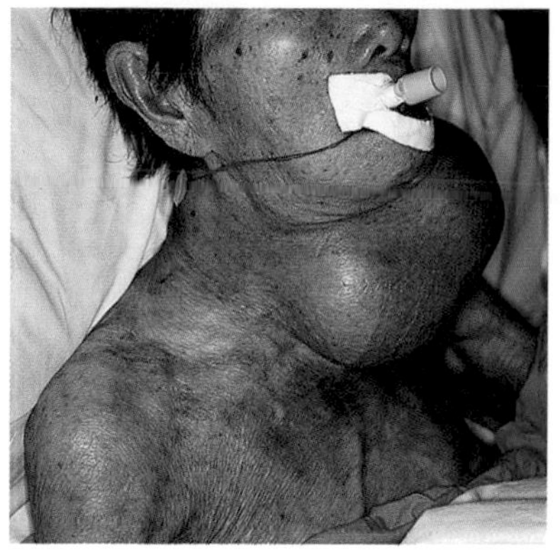

7. **This patient has been intubated for planned neck surgery.**

a. What is the diagnosis?
b. What clinical features would raise the suspicion of an underlying thyroid malignancy?
c. What are the indications for surgery in a patient with thyrotoxicosis?

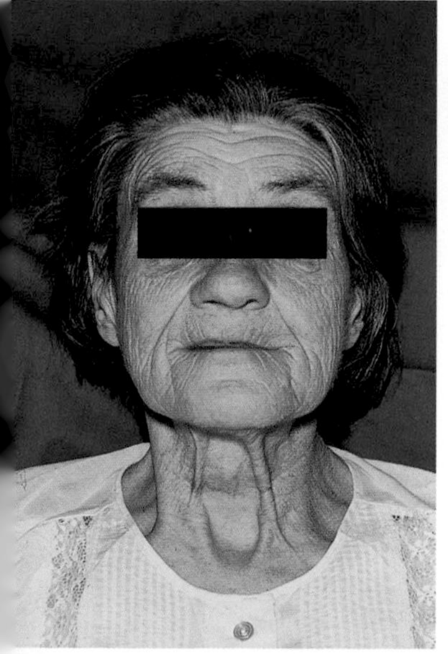

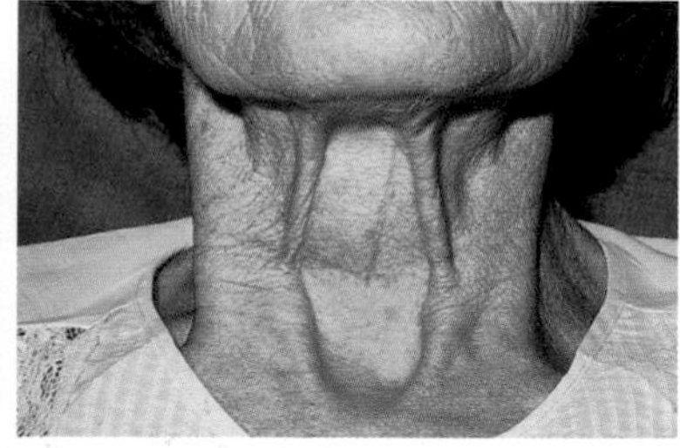

8. **This elderly lady's main complaint was of lethargy.**

a. Why has this patient developed hypothyroidism?
b. How can the general thyroid status of a patient be assessed?
c. How should patients with hypothyroidism be managed?

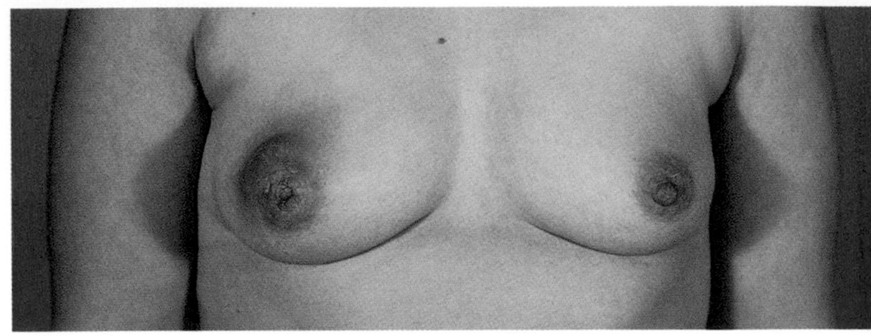

9. **This middle-aged lady presented with a painful swelling in her right breast.**

a. What is the diagnosis?
b. What risk factor is associated with periductal mastitis and non-lactational breast abscess formation?
c. What is the appropriate treatment for this condition?

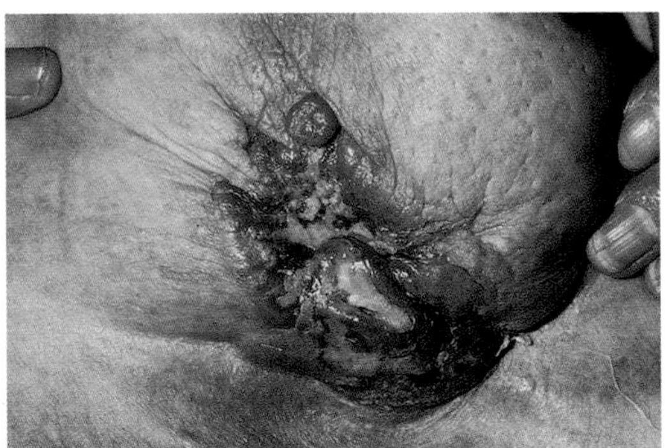

10. **This elderly lady had had an ulcerating lesion of her breast for 9 months prior to presentation.**

a. What is the diagnosis?
b. What percentage of breast cancers have a genetic predisposition?
c. What pointers are there to an inherited disposition?
d. What factors adversely affect outcome in patients with breast cancer?

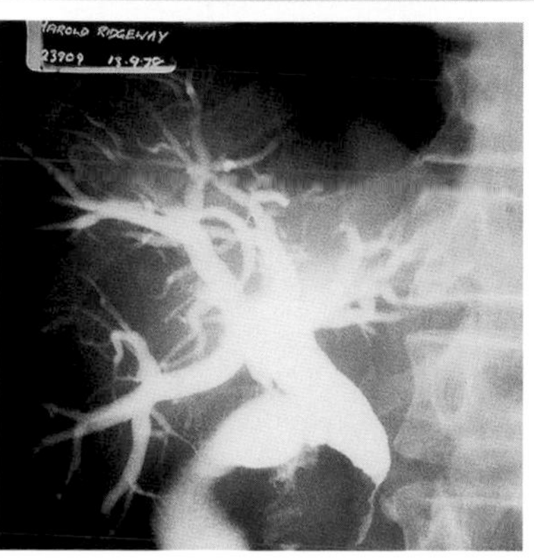

A

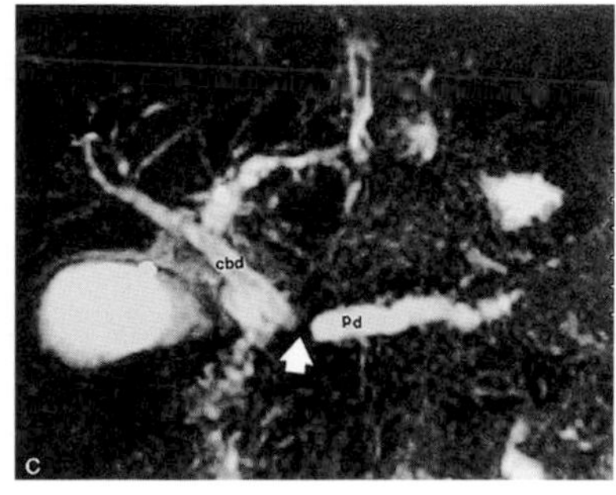

B

11. These investigations were undertaken in an elderly man who presented with jaundice.

a. What are these investigations?
b. What abnormality do they demonstrate?
c. What further investigations should be undertaken?
d. What are the treatment options?

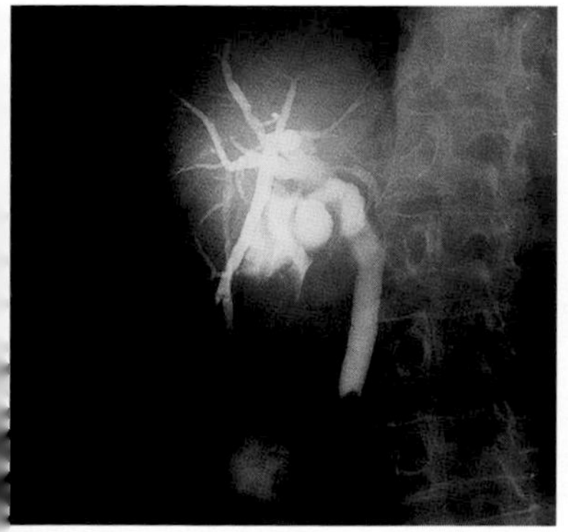

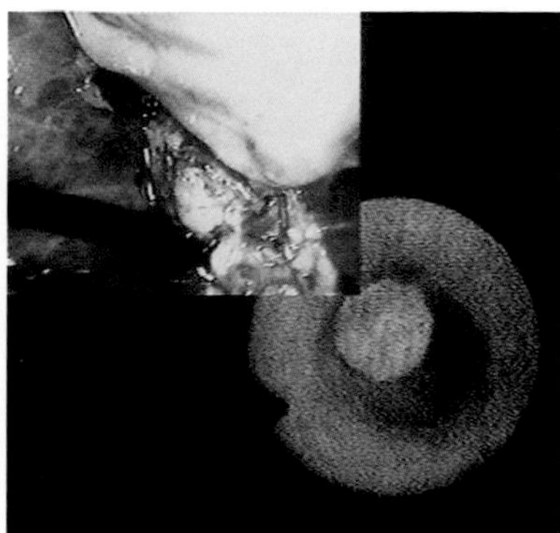

12. These images were obtained during the course of an operation.

a. What does the intraoperative cholangiogram demonstrate?
b. What does the intraoperative photograph show?
c. What is the therapeutic strategy?
d. What options are available if the ductal calculus cannot be retrieved by laparoscopic means?

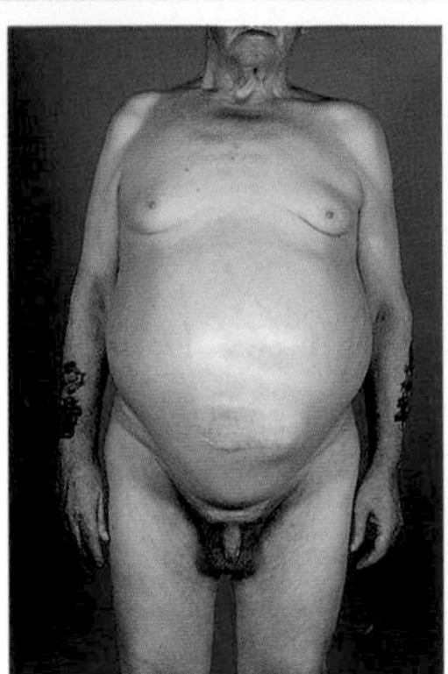

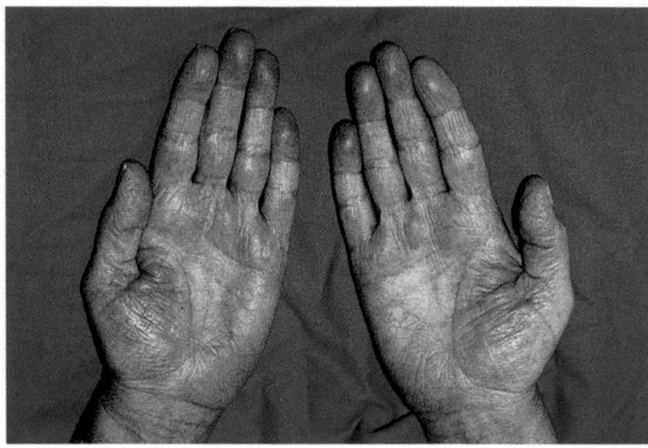

13. **This patient had a longstanding history of chronic liver disease.**

a. What clinical features of liver cirrhosis are seen in this patient?
b. What other clinical features should be looked for in a patient with known liver cirrhosis?
c. What are the principal complications of portal hypertension?
d. What are the treatment options for portal hypertension?

14. **This lady has a long-standing history of abdominal pain**

a. What is the diagnosis?
b. What investigations should be considered before planning the management strategy?
c. What are the available methods of treatment for pancreatic pseudocysts?

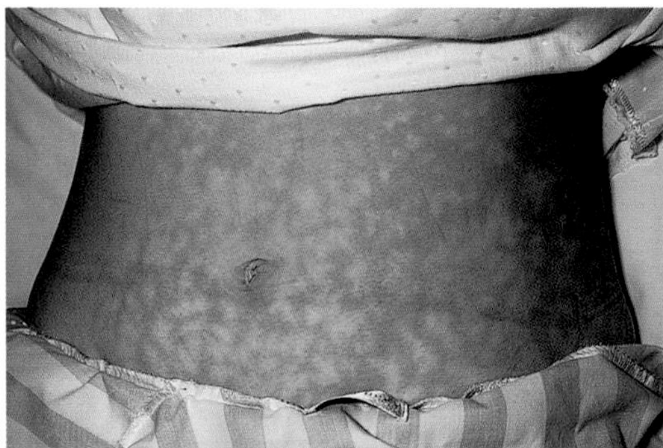

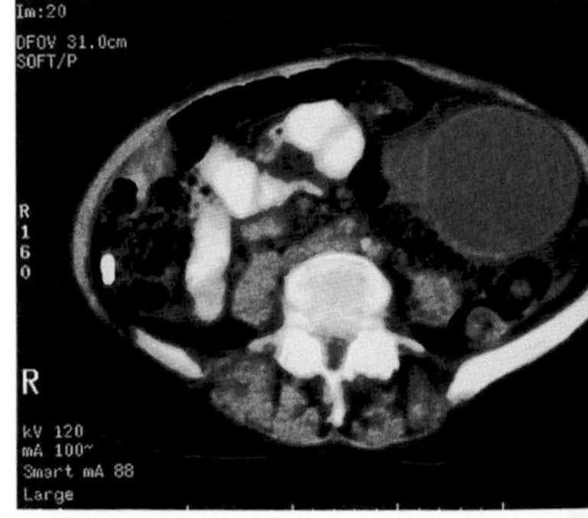

15. This patient had noted a progressive swelling at the site of a previous midline abdominal wound.

a. What is the diagnosis?
b. What are the risk factors for developing such a condition?
c. What is the recommended treatment?
d. What are the risks of recurrence?

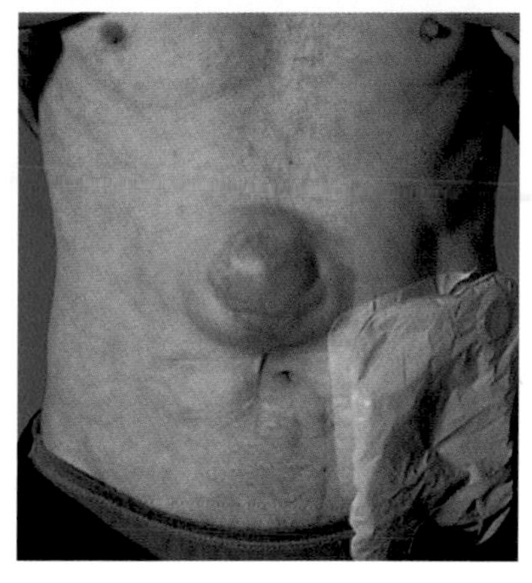

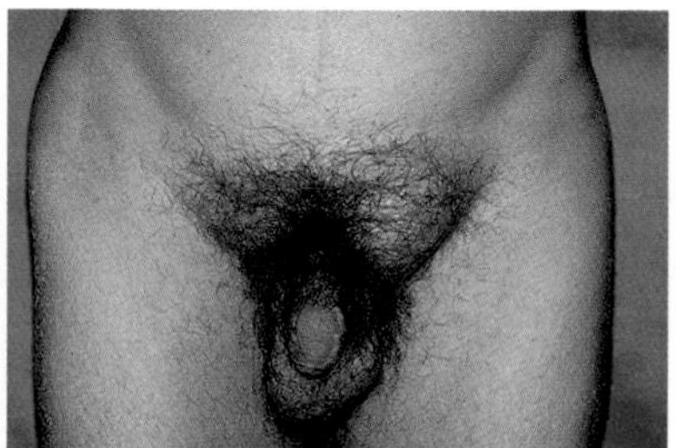

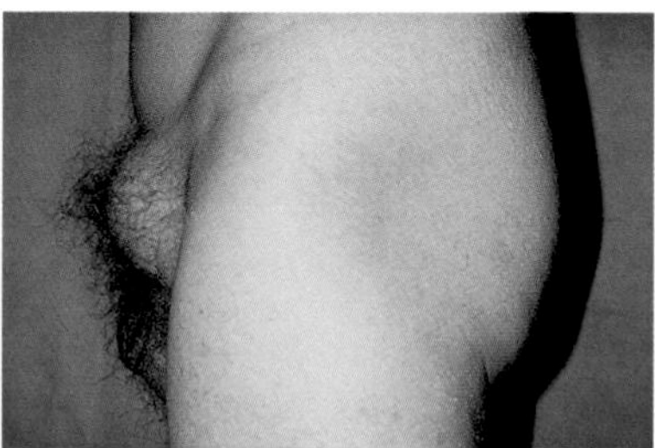

16. This man had a 6-month history of a painful left groin swelling.

a. What is the diagnosis?
b. What is the difference in the anatomical course of an indirect and a direct inguinal hernia?
c. What is the operation most commonly undertaken to repair an inguinal hernia?
d. What is the risk of recurrence after repair of an inguinal hernia?

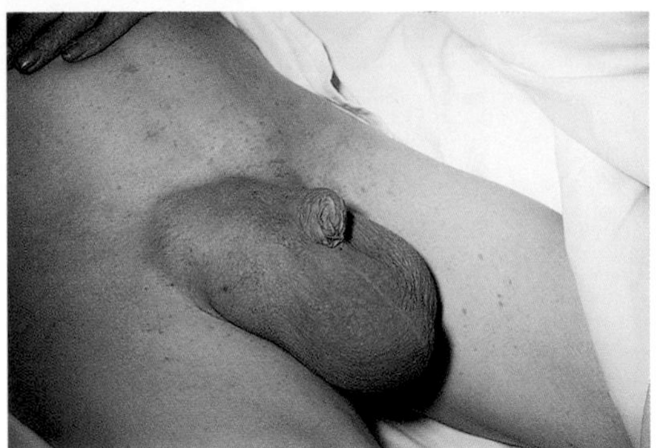

17. **This patient presented with a scrotal swelling.**

a. What is the differential diagnosis of this scrotal swelling?
b. What is the risk of malignancy associated with a hydrocele?
c. What investigations should be undertaken?
d. What is the treatment for a hydrocele?

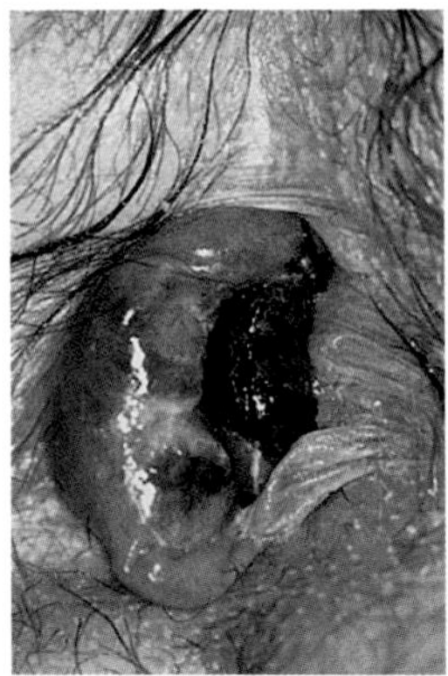

A

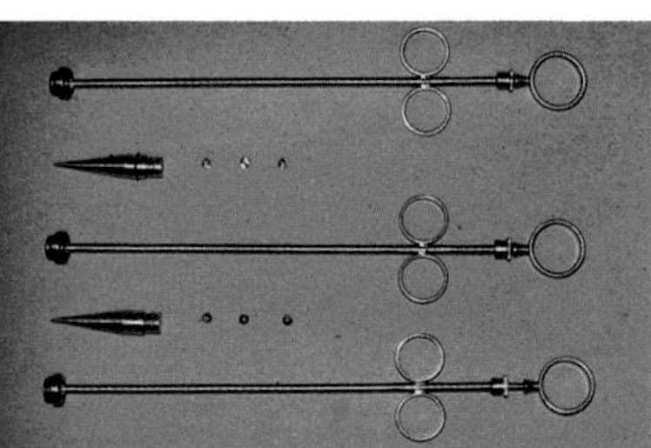

B

18. **This abnormality was seen on inspection of the anus.**

a. What is the condition shown in Figure A?
b. What are the instruments shown in Figure B?
c. What are the treatment options for symptomatic haemorrhoids?

19. **This patient presented acutely with perineal pain.**

a. What is the diagnosis?
b. What is the source of the infection?
c. How should this lesion be managed?
d. What may subsequently develop after drainage of a perianal abscess?

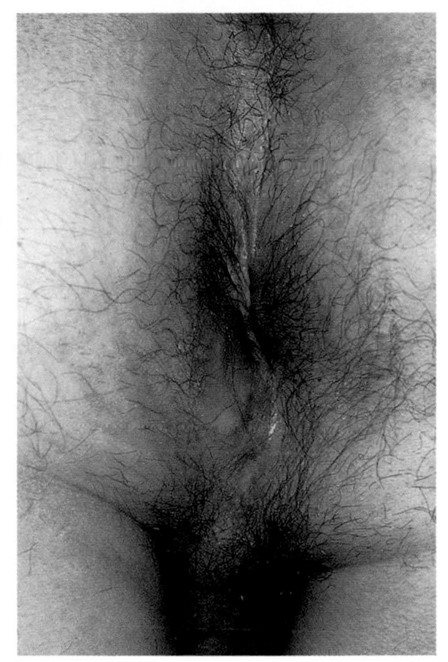

20. **This patient presented with intermittent anal discharge.**

a. What is demonstrated in this illustration?
b. How can these abnormalities be classified?
c. How can this condition be investigated?
d. How should such lesions be treated?

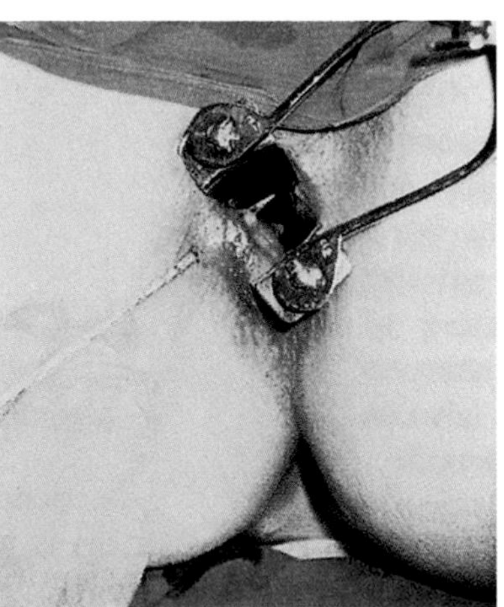

21. This condition affects the natal cleft

a. What is the diagnosis?
b. How might the patient present?
c. What is the appropriate management of this condition?

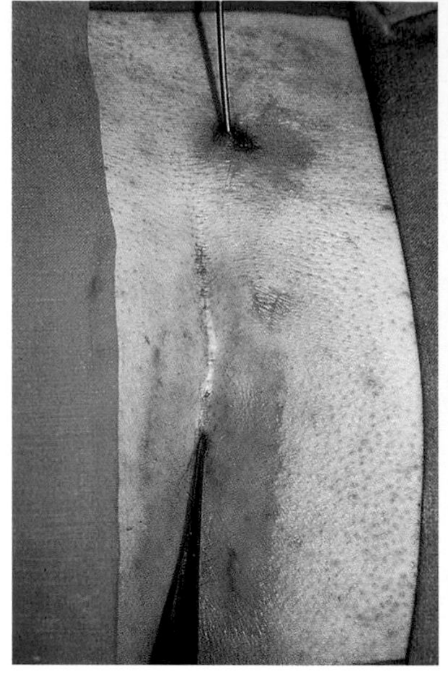

22. This lesion required surgical treatment.

a. What is the diagnosis?
b. Who characteristically gets this condition?
c. What is the management of this condition?

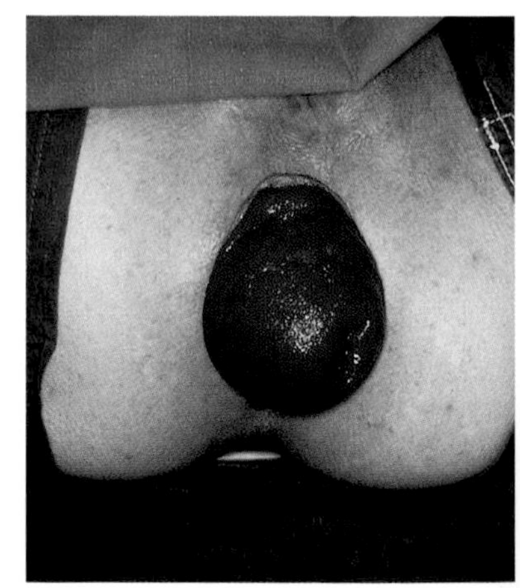

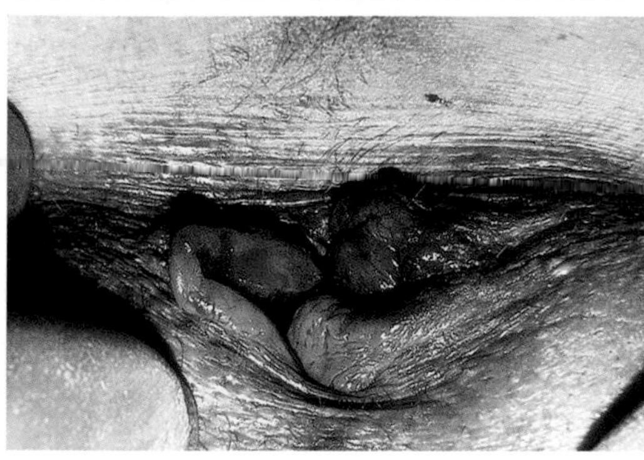

23. This anal lesion was hard on palpation.

a. What is the lesion?
b. What is the usual cell type of this malignancy?
c. What is the management of this lesion?

24. This stoma was exposed after removal of an appliance from the anterior abdominal wall.

a. What is this stoma likely to be?
b. What is the abnormality seen on the stoma?
c. What are the complications associated with such a stoma?
d. Other than small bowel contents, what other material could drain from a similar stoma?

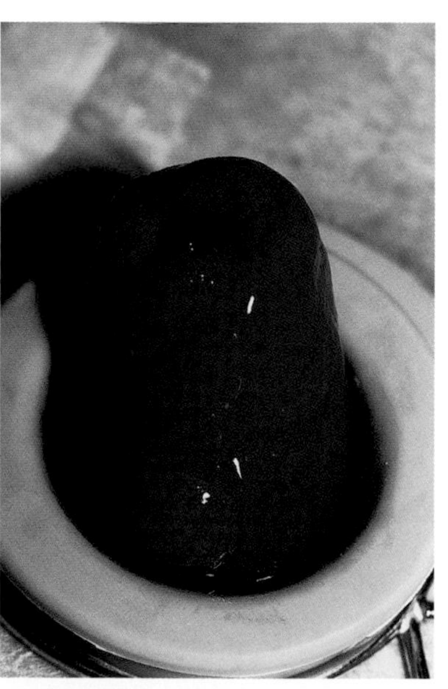

25. This patient has a painful right foot.

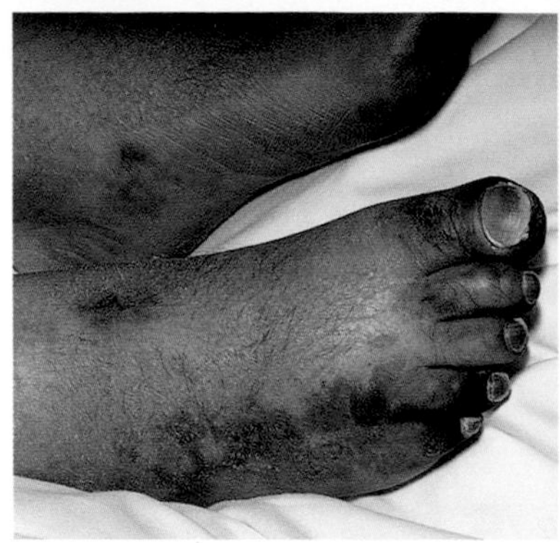

a. What is the diagnosis?
b. What is the immediate management?
c. What definitive surgical intervention could be considered?
d. What is the likely prognosis?

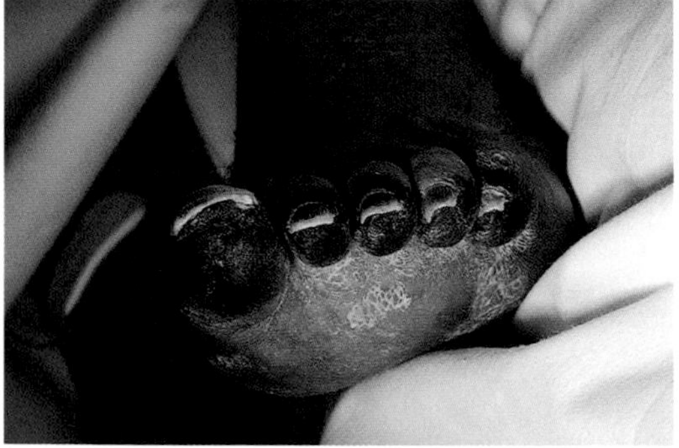

26. This patient presented to a vascular clinic.

a. What is the diagnosis?
b. What complication can affect this condition?
c. What is the usual causal organism?
d. What is the treatment for this complicated condition?

27. This male patient was admitted electively to hospital for scheduled surgery.

a. What is the diagnosis?
b. What is the likely clinical presentation?
c. What is the treatment of this condition?

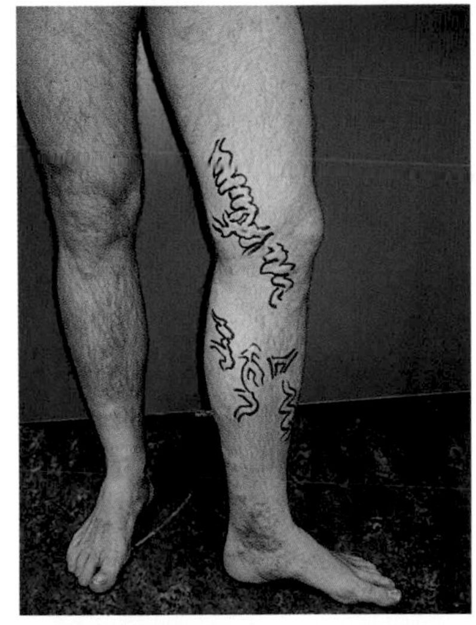

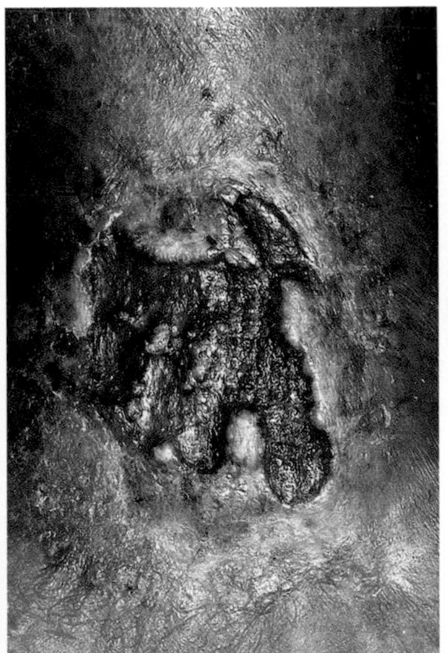

A

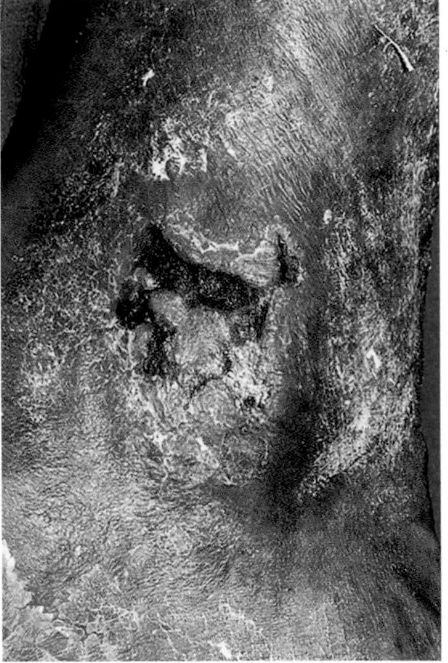

B

28. This patient has long-standing untreated varicose veins.

a. What is the diagnosis?
b. What other skin changes may be seen with this condition?
c. Where is the typical site of such a lesion?
d. What is the management of these lesions?

29. This patient has undergone breast surgery.

a. What is the diagnosis?
b. What is characteristic of the type of swelling?
c. What is the management of such a condition?

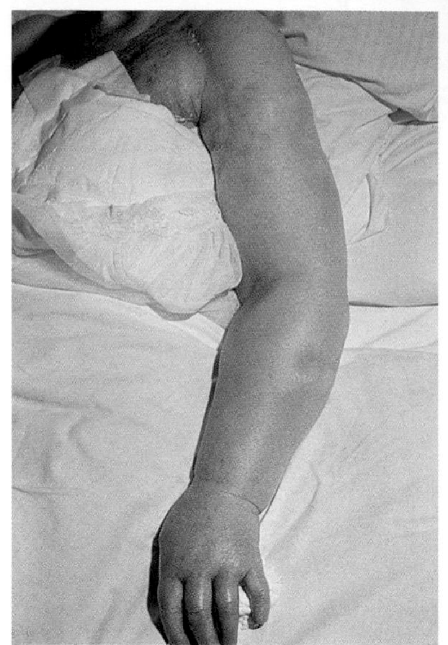

Answers

1. *a.* Basal cell carcinoma. This lesion most commonly occurs in patients with fair dry skin constantly exposed to sunlight.
b. The majority of lesions occur on the face above the line joining the angle of the mouth and the lobe of the ear, but no part of the skin is exempt.
c. The lesion spreads superficially or deeply. Spread may be so extensive as to destroy the nose and eyes and erode through the skull, but the tumour rarely metastasizes.
d. If the diagnosis is uncertain an incision biopsy or scraping for cytology can be confirmatory. Excision, with 5 mm of normal skin is the treatment of choice for most patients. Superficial radiotherapy is effective but should be reserved for biopsy proven lesions once surgery is contraindicated. Superficial basal cell carcinomas can be treated with curettage and cautery, cryotherapy, topical 5-fluorouracil or photodynamic therapy.

2. *a.* Squamous cell carcinoma.
b. Long-term ultraviolet radiation is an immunosuppressant of the skin and is the main aetiological factor in these malignant tumours of keratinocytes.
c. Surgical excision with a 5 mm margin. As with basal cell carcinoma, radiotherapy can be used in selected cases. Follow-up is advised to assess for local recurrence, evidence of metastases and further primary tumours.

3. *a.* Malignant melanoma.
b.
- Lentigo maligna (Hutchinson's freckle) – the least malignant type
- Superficial spreading – the commonest form of melanoma
- Nodular melanoma – this is the form shown in the figure and is the most ominous type
- Acral lentiginous – these are melanomas occurring on the palms of the hands, soles of the feet and under the nails (subungual melanoma)
- Amelanotic – a special form of nodular melanoma with a worse prognosis

c. Only surgical excision is effective. A 3 cm clearance is recommended for tumours greater than 1 mm thick. Tumours less than 1 mm thick can be removed with a 1 cm clearance. Palpable lymph nodes should always be removed by radical block dissection.
d. The prognosis is excellent for those tumours less than 1 mm thick (over 90% survive 5 years), but becomes less good with thicker tumours. The 5 year survival of patients with tumours more than 3.5 mm thick is about 50%.

4. *a.* Figure A shows a superficial partial-thickness burn (sometimes referred to as a first-degree burn). Figure B shows a deep partial-thickness burn (often referred to as a second-degree burn). A full-thickness burn can be described as a third-degree burn.

b. A superficial partial-thickness burn will heal completely with no residual scarring usually within 3 weeks. With a deep partial-thickness burn, fewer epithelial elements survive and therefore the attenuated surviving dermis heals with the production of disfiguring hypertrophic scars.

c. Fires kill more people by asphyxia than by burns and therefore the first medical priority is management of the airway and breathing. The main threat to the upper airway occurs when laryngeal oedema develops following direct thermal injury caused by the inhalation of flame, hot gases or steam. Endotracheal intubation or emergency tracheostomy may be required and oxygen should be administered.

d. Adults with 15% and children with 10% body involvement lose sufficient fluid to be at risk of hypovolemic shock. Most fluid is lost in the first 12 h but substantial fluid loss is continued for at least another 36 h. Since much of the fluid lost is essentially plasma, the main type of fluid replacement should be a plasma substitute, with the remainder consisting of isotonic electrolyte solution. Fluid balance must be monitored according to pulse, blood pressure and urine output.

e. Prevention of infection after skin grafting to minimize the likelihood of graft failure and regrafting, as this increases the likelihood of developing hypertrophic scars. Intensive efforts have also been made using physiotherapy, splinting and compression bandaging to lessen the effects of contractures and facilitate joint movement.

5. *a.* Necrotizing fascitis (Fournier's gangrene). This is an invasive infection that spreads quickly and causes necrosis of fat and fascia with overlying secondary necrosis of skin.

b. Streptococci and anaerobes are the most likely causative organisms.

c. Wide surgical debridement. The wound should be left open for secondary closure. Parenteral antibiotics, including penicillin and metronidazole, should be prescribed after samples have been taken for culture and sensitivity.

6. *a.* Parotid tumour. Pleomorphic adenoma is by far the most common neoplasm of salivary gland origin. It is also the most common cause of a lump in the parotid or submandibular gland.

b. Pleomorphic adenoma of the parotid classically presents as a very slow-growing, painless lump.

c. Treatment of pleomorphic adenoma is by excision. For superficial lesions, this is usually by superficial parotidectomy, which involves excision of all glandular tissue superficial to the plane of the facial nerve.

d. Damage to branches of the facial nerve.

7. *a.* Thyroid goitre. This term is used to describe any generalized enlargement of the thyroid. When the condition is endemic, iodine insufficiency is the usual cause. These goitres are often asymmetrical and soft to palpation. Although they can reach enormous size, endemic goitres cause surprisingly few symptoms and the patient is usually euthyroid. Anaplastic carcinomas may also cause fairly large thyroid swellings in elderly patients. The uncommon lymphomas of the thyroid also present with diffuse thyroid enlargement. In Graves disease (primary hyperthyroidism) there is usually a degree of smooth thyroid enlargement; however, this is rarely the presenting feature. Similarly, in Hashimoto's thyroiditis, the thyroid may be enlarged but firmer and nodular on palpation. Multinodular goitre may present with a significant neck swelling.

b. A rapidly enlarging hard thyroid mass in an elderly patient may be due to an underlying malignancy. There may be symptoms suggesting invasion into nearby structures, such as hoarseness if there is recurrent laryngeal nerve involvement, or stridor, particularly at night, if there is tracheal displacement or compression.

c.
- Surgery is a quick and effective cure when long-term drug therapy with carbimazole is undesirable
- It is often the best treatment for Graves disease, particularly in young patients
- Failure of antithyroid drugs or if radioiodine is unsuitable, e.g. in females of childbearing age
- For multinodular goitre where response to drug treatment is unreliable
- Toxic solitary nodules are best excised

8. *a.* This patient has had previous thyroid surgery. Hypothyroidism is a late complication in up to 25% of patients after subtotal thyroidectomy for thyrotoxicosis and is inevitable after total thyroidectomy for carcinoma.

b. Clinically a patient with hypothyroidism may present with tiredness, malaise, constipation, depression or weight gain. On physical examination, the patient may have puffy eyes, dry skin and coarse hair. They may have hoarseness and a bradycardia. Estimations of serum thyroxine (T_4) and thyroid stimulating hormone (TSH) should be measured. Tri-iodothyronine (T_3) concentrations do not discriminate reliably between euthyroid and hypothyroid patients and should not be measured routinely.

c. Hypothyroidism should be treated with thyroxine. It is customary to start with a dose of 50 mg per day for 3 weeks increasing thereafter to 100 mg per day for a further 3 weeks and finally to 150 mg per day if required. The correct dose of thyroxine is that which restores serum TSH to normal. Patients feel better within 2–3 weeks. Reduction in weight and periorbital puffiness occurs quickly, but the restoration of skin and hair texture and resolution of any effusions may take 3–6 months.

9. *a.* Breast abscess.

b. Smoking is an important aetiological factor in 90% of women who present with periductal mastitis or its complications. It is thought that substances in cigarette smoke either directly or indirectly damage the subareolar breast ducts and the damaged tissue then becomes infected by either aerobic or anaerobic organisms. Initial presentation may be with periareolar inflammation, with or without an associated mass, or with an established abscess.

c. Treatment for periductal mastitis is with antibiotics. Abscesses are managed by aspiration or incision and drainage. Following drainage of a non-lactational breast abscess, up to a third of patients develop a mammary duct fistula. Recurrent episodes of periareolar infection require excision of the diseased ducts.

10. *a.* Breast carcinoma.

b. Up to 10% of breast cancers in Western society are due to a genetic predisposition. The genetic contribution is mainly through single genes inherited as autosomal dominant but with limited penetrance. Not all gene carriers develop breast cancer. Four human breast cancer genes have been identified: *BRCA1, BRCA2, p53* and *PTEN*. In breast cancer families there is also an increased risk of other tumours, notably ovarian cancer.

c. A first-degree relative who develops breast cancer under the age of 40 years, numerous family relatives with breast cancer or a close family relative who has had ovarian cancer. Options for high-risk women include regular screening, prevention using tamoxifen or prophylactic bilateral mastectomy.

d. The most important prognostic factor is lymph node status. Other factors that adversely affect outcome are the presence of metastases, tumour grade, oestrogen receptor status, vascular or lymphatic invasion by tumour and evidence of extensive angiogenesis. It is possible to combine independent prognostic factors to form an index that allows the identification of groups of patients with different prognoses. The Nottingham prognostic index is the most widely used and is calculated as follows: NPI = $(0.2 \times \text{size (cm)})$ + score lymph node stage (1–3) + score of grade (1–3).

11. *a.* Both are cholangiograms. Figure A may represent a percutaneous transhepatic cholangiogram or an endoscopic retrograde cholangiogram after removal of the endoscope. Figure B is the result of a magnetic resonance cholangiopancreatogram (MRCP).

b. Both images show obstruction of the distal common bile duct, most probably due to a pancreatic neoplasm.

c. A CT scan may demonstrate a mass lesion in the head of the pancreas. Assessment for resectability is determined by excluding local vascular invasion and distant metastases. Other modalities that may be used in the staging of patients with pancreatic cancer include endoscopic ultrasound and laparoscopy with laparoscopic ultrasonography.

d. Curative treatment entails pancreaticoduodenectomy (Whipple's procedure). The objective of palliative treatment is to relieve jaundice, pruritus, pain and duodenal obstruction. Insertion of a prosthetic stent either endoscopically or radiologically via the percutaneous transhepatic route will relieve jaundice. Median survival for patients with unresectable pancreatic cancer is approximately 8 months.

12. *a.* The cholangiogram shows a calculus in the distal common bile duct.
b. A mobile calculus visualized by laparoscopic choledochoscopy.
c. Under direct vision using the choledochoscope, a wire basket is inserted down the operating channel of the choledochoscope and the calculus is retrieved with a basket and removed.
d. Conversion to an open procedure with open exploration of the common bile duct or early postoperative ERCP with sphincterotomy and stone retrieval.

13. *a.* Palmar erythema – it is of limited diagnostic value as it occurs in many other conditions associated with a hyperdynamic circulation as well as in some normal people. Endocrine changes are noted, namely loss of male hair distribution, testicular atrophy and gynaecomastia. Ascites is due to a combination of liver failure and portal hypertension and signifies advanced disease.
b. Mild jaundice may be due to a failure to excrete bilirubin. Spider telangiectasia are due to associated arteriolar changes and comprise a central arteriole from which small vessels radiate. Hepatomegaly may be found in early cirrhosis but progressive fibrosis gradually reduces the liver size as the disease progresses. Splenomegaly, collateral vessel formation and fetor hepaticus are features of portal hypertension. Non-specific features of chronic liver disease include pigmentation, finger clubbing and Dupuytren's contracture.
c. Variceal bleeding and ascites.
d. Bleeding oesophageal varices can usually be controlled by endoscopic variceal ligation or injection sclerotherapy. Oesophageal tamponade may be necessary in the acute setting if endoscopic variceal ligation or injection sclerotherapy is not available. Oesophageal transection may be required if endoscopic therapy fails. Spironolactone is the diuretic of choice for management of ascites. Transjugular intrahepatic portosystemic shunt (TIPSS) may be indicated in patients with portal hypertension but can be complicated by hepatic encephalopathy. Chronic liver failure due to cirrhosis can be treated by orthotopic liver transplantation.

14. *a.* Chronic pancreatitis with erythema ab igne due to chronic use of a hot water bottle and evidence of a pancreatic pseudocyst on CT scan. The development of a pancreatic pseudocyst may be associated with acute pancreatitis (requires 4 or more weeks from the onset of acute pancreatitis; prior to this the abnormality is known as an acute fluid collection) or chronic pancreatitis.

b. An ERCP may be helpful to delineate the pancreatic duct morphology and may show communication between the pancreatic duct and the pseudocyst. Endoscopic ultrasound may be useful to assess the suitability for transmural endoscopic drainage.

c. Endoscopic drainage of pseudocysts can be performed transpapillary or trans-murally through the stomach or duodenum depending on the site of the pseudocyst. Only cysts which are clearly bulging in to the bowel lumen and with a wall thickness of less than 10 mm are suitable for endoscopic transmural drainage. Surgical drainage is achieved by anastomosing the stomach, duodenum or a Roux-en-Y limb of jejunum to the most dependent part of the pseudocyst wall. Traditionally, surgical intervention has been undertaken at an open operation; however, more recently laparoscopic approaches have been described.

15. *a.* Incisional hernia.

b. Poor surgical technique, wound infection, obesity, jaundice, steroid therapy and postoperative chest infection are important predisposing factors.

c. Surgical repair is recommended even for asymptomatic patients. At operation the sac can be invaginated and, if the defect is small, the edges can be repaired by an overlapping Mayo-type repair. Otherwise a synthetic mesh should be used.

d. Small incisional hernias have a recurrence rate of 2–5%, whereas larger incisional hernias have a recurrence rate of 10–20%.

16. *a.* Inguinal hernia.

b. An indirect inguinal hernia leaves the abdomen via the deep (internal) inguinal ring lateral to the inferior epigastric vessels and travels along the inguinal canal to emerge at the superficial (external) inguinal ring above and medial to the pubic tubercle. The coverings are the attenuated layers of the spermatic cord. A direct inguinal hernia protrudes directly through the transversalis fascia of the posterior wall of the inguinal canal, medial to the inferior epigastric vessels, and is not covered by layers of the spermatic cord.

c. An open Lichtenstein tension-free repair. Laparoscopic inguinal hernia repair is particularly useful in patients with recurrent or bilateral inguinal hernias.

d. Recurrence rates in specialist units approach 0%; however, in most general surgical series the reported recurrence rate is 1–5%.

17. *a.* Hydrocele, epididymal cyst, testicular tumour, epididymo-orchitis, varicocele or an indirect inguinal hernia.

b. In adults, 10% of hydroceles are associated with an underlying testicular tumour.

c. Blood tumour markers and an ultrasound scan of the scrotum should be undertaken to exclude an underlying testicular neoplasm.

d. Aspiration of fluid is commonly associated with recollection of fluid. Injection of a sclerosant following aspiration may prevent reaccumulation but the treatment of choice is surgery. The tunica vaginalis can be partially excised and everted behind the epididymis if it is thin-walled (Jaboulay's operation). Alternatively, the tunica vaginalis can be completely excised if it is thick-walled. Meticulous haemostasis is particularly important to prevent postoperative scrotal haematoma or haematocele formation.

18. *a.* Thrombosed and prolapsed haemorrhoids.

b. They are rubber band applicators.

c. Many patients will require no treatment as symptoms are minor and intermittent. Constipation should be avoided and medication may be required to regulate bowel habit. A number of non-operative approaches for treatment are available, which include rubber band ligation to strangulate the haemorrhoids, submucosal injection of sclerosant or application of heat using infrared photocoagulation. All these procedures can be performed in the outpatient department. Traditional haemorrhoidectomy involves total removal of the haemorrhoidal mass and securing of haemostasis. The wound can be left open or can be closed. Recently a different surgical approach using a circular stapler has been developed. This technique aims to divide the mucosa and haemorrhoidal cushions above the dentate line in order to transect the feeding vessels and hitch up the stretched supporting tissue. Symptomatic relief of thrombosed or strangulated haemorrhoids is often achieved by bed rest and by applying ice packs and local anaesthetic gel. Acute haemorrhoidectomy under antibiotic cover provides definitive management for both thrombosed and strangulated haemorrhoids but carries a higher risk of complications.

19. *a.* Recurrent perianal abscess.

b. A perianal abscess is thought to develop when pus tracks inferiorly from infection arising in the anal glands.

c. Diabetes or any other cause of immune deficiency should be excluded. If suppuration has occurred, the abscess should be drained. An elliptical or cruciate incision should be performed, a swab of pus should be sent for bacteriological culture, any loculi within the cavity should be broken down and the cavity should be packed loosely to allow healing from the base by secondary intention. Antibiotics are only indicated if there is spreading cellulitis.

d. A significant number of patients develop an anal fistula, which may require further investigation and treatment.

20. *a.* An anal fistula.

b. The fistulous track can be intersphincteric, trans-sphincteric or suprasphincteric.

c. Digital palpation may reveal induration between the external orifice and the anal canal in keeping with the subcutaneous track. Patients require rigid sigmoidoscopy or proctoscopy and often require examination under anaesthetic.

d. Management is determined by the course of the fistulous tract. Low fistula can be simply laid open and allowed to heal by secondary intention. However where a significant proportion of the internal and/or external sphincter is involved, laying open the tract can result in faecal incontinence. In such complex cases, a seton suture or sloop can be inserted into the fistulous tract to allow the fistula to drain. The seton suture or sloop will gradually cut out through the sphincters, allowing them to heal behind the seton. High suprasphincteric anal fistula may require complex surgical intervention and occasionally formation of a defunctioning colostomy may be necessary.

21. *a.* Pilonidal sinus.

b. Typical presenting features are of recurrent episodes of pain, tenderness and purulent discharge. Superadded infection may result in formation of a pilonidal abscess with a fluctuant mass and inflammation and induration of the surrounding skin.

c. A pilonidal abscess requires surgical drainage. A chronic pilonidal sinus can be laid open and the wound allowed to heal by secondary intention. Simple superficial pilonidal disease may be excised and closed primarily with sutures.

22. *a.* Rectal prolapse.

b. Rectal prolapse is mainly seen in young children and in the elderly. In childhood, rectal prolapse usually occurs around the age of 2 years during toilet training. In the elderly rectal prolapse is either remarkably well tolerated or else concealed.

c. Children should be given a high-fibre diet and taught not to strain during defaecation. A high-fibre diet makes little difference to the problem in the elderly since the anatomical defect will never recover spontaneously. If the prolapse occurs on standing or if incontinence develops, the patient is likely to require surgical treatment. The abdominal operations include suture fixation rectopexy and resection rectopexy. The popular perineal procedures include Delorme's operation and Altemeirer's procedure.

23. *a.* Anal cancer.

b. 80% of anal cancer is squamous cell carcinoma and approximately 10% of tumours are adenocarcinoma. Other rarer tumours include melanoma, lymphoma and sarcoma.

c. Investigations should include an examination under anaesthesia with sigmoidoscopy and tissue biopsy. Histological confirmation of the diagnosis allows appropriate further treatment. Radiotherapy is the current standard treatment for squamous cell cancer, combined with chemotherapy using 5-fluorouracil and mitomycin C. Surgery may play a part in advanced disease or in very early tumours that can be completely excised. The overall 5-year survival rate is approximately 60%.

24. *a.* An ilesotomy, as a spout has been fashioned.
b. There is ulceration of the stoma due to underlying Crohn's disease.
c. Complications associated with an ileostomy include skin erosion if a stoma bag is not fitted correctly, prolapse of the small bowel, parastomal hernia formation, retraction of the stoma, stenosis of the stomal orifice and parastomal fistula formation. The latter complication is more likely if the underlying diagnosis is Crohn's disease.
d. Urine could drain from an ileal conduit. This may be fashioned if the urinary bladder is resected and the ureters are then drained into an isolated segment of small bowel, which is brought out as a spout in a similar fashion to an end-ileostomy.

25. *a.* This patient has critical limb ischaemia due to acute thrombosis/occlusion of pre-existing atherosclerotic vessels. There is marked discoloration of the toes and forefoot, with absent pedal pulses.
b. The case should be discussed with a vascular surgeon. An intravenous bolus of heparin should be administered to limit propagation of thrombus. If there has been sudden loss of sensation, loss of active movement or pain on passive movement when the calf muscles are squeezed, it would suggest a threatened limb and in these circumstances an urgent embolectomy or thrombectomy should be considered. In a non-threatened limb, a period of medical optimization on heparin therapy may lead to spontaneous improvement. Thrombolysis may be attempted in these circumstances.
c. Assessment should be undertaken to determine if percutaneous transluminal balloon angioplasty would be appropriate or whether the patient requires arterial surgical reconstruction. It is important to determine on angiography the level of occlusion and whether there is adequate distal run-off. Arterial surgical reconstruction may require femoral–popliteal bypass or femoral–distal bypass.
d. Surgical reconstruction is associated with a mortality rate of 1–5%. In-hospital mortality for patients requiring major limb amputation is approximately 10–20%.

26. *a.* Gangrene of the toes. Gangrene is the presence of dead tissue and is the end stage of peripheral vascular disease.
b. Superadded infection. Dry gangrene occurs when dead tissue mummifies without infection. This usually results in the affected area separating from the healthy tissues spontaneously (autoamputation). If the necrotic area becomes infected, the gangrene is described as 'wet gangrene' and will spread proximally and cause systemic upset.
c. Clostridia.
d. Urgent treatment is required. Revascularization of the ischaemic limb combined with antibiotics may be successful; however, debridement or amputation is often required.

27. *a.* Varicose veins.

b. The most common presenting feature is the cosmetic appearance of the varicosities. Symptoms include heaviness and aching of the limbs and ankle swelling.

c. Conservative treatment involves elastic compression stockings, weight reduction, regular exercise and avoidance of prolonged standing. The aim of injection sclerotherapy is to produce a sterile chemical inflammation of the vein, which is kept empty by compression. This causes thrombosis and obliteration of the vessel lumen and is suitable for small varicosities below the knee or for recurrent varicose veins following primary surgery. Varicose vein surgery aims to remove the varicosities and disconnect incompetent perforators between the deep and superficial veins to prevent further varicosities from developing. For patients with long saphenous vein disease, the saphenofemoral junction is ligated flush with the femoral vein. In patients with short saphenous disease the saphenopopliteal junction is dealt with in a similar fashion. The long saphenous vein in the thigh may be stripped from the groin to the knee and the remaining varicosities are then avulsed through multiple tiny stab incisions.

28. *a.* Chronic venous ulceration. This is the end result of chronic venous insufficiency.

b. Chronic venous hypertension causes skin changes such as lipodermatosclerosis, pigmentation and eczematous change. Oedema is common but eventually fibrosis may produce scar tissue around the ankle with oedema proximally.

c. The most common site is over the medial or lateral malleolus and the ulcer is often precipitated by minor trauma.

d. It is important to exclude deep vein occlusion. The 'four-layer bandage' is popular and often results in good healing. Figure B shows the dramatic healing of the ulcer after 2 weeks intensive treatment with compression bandaging. Surgical intervention may be required to treat the underlying varicose veins and calf perforators. Occasionally, skin grafting may be required to speed up ulcer healing.

29. *a.* Secondary limb lymphoedema. This occurs when there is obstruction of the lymphatic drainage of the limb, which in this case has been caused by obliteration of the axillary lymphatics due to surgery but may be due to malignant infiltration of the axillary lymph nodes or recurrent infection.

b. The oedema is persistent and associated with tissue fibrosis, giving a classical 'non-pitting' oedema.

c. Lymphodema is a clinical diagnosis and investigation is not required. The principal of management is initial elevation of the limb. Intermittent pneumatic compression devices and regular massage are often useful; however, the mainstay of therapy is graduated compression hosiery. Diuretics are not beneficial and more often cause troublesome side effects.

Index

Page numbers in *italics* refer to questions and answers.

H

I

J

K

L

M

N

O

P

R

S

T

U

V

W

X

Z